Migrating for
Medical Marijuana

Migrating for Medical Marijuana

Pioneers in a New Frontier of Treatment

TRACY FERRELL

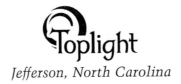

Jefferson, North Carolina

LIBRARY OF CONGRESS CATALOGUING-IN-PUBLICATION DATA

Names: Ferrell, Tracy, 1970– author.
Title: Migrating for medical marijuana : pioneers in a new frontier
of treatment / Tracy Ferrell.
Description: Jefferson, North Carolina : Toplight, 2019 |
Includes bibliographical references and index.
Identifiers: LCCN 2019033992 | ISBN 9781476678597 (softcover : acid free paper) ∞ |
ISBN 9781476637235 (ebook)
Subjects: LCSH: Marijuana—Therapeutic use—Colorado. | Marijuana—Physiological
effect. | Marijuana—Law and legislation—Colorado. | Travel.
Classification: LCC RM666.C266 F47 2019 | DDC 615.3/23648—dc23
LC record available at https://lccn.loc.gov/2019033992

BRITISH LIBRARY CATALOGUING DATA ARE AVAILABLE

ISBN (print) 978-1-4766-7859-7
ISBN (ebook) 978-1-4766-3723-5

Front cover images © 2019 Shutterstock

Printed in the United States of America

Toplight is an imprint of McFarland & Company, Inc., Publishers

Box 611, Jefferson, North Carolina 28640
www.toplightbooks.com

To the thousands of patients and their families using cannabis to treat their ailments, especially those who were kind enough to speak with me for this book. Your bravery in facing down the law and the medical establishment to find a treatment or cure is an inspiration.

You cannot make a war against drugs without knowing that, doing so, you are making a war against people.—Ruth Driefus, former president of the Swiss Confederation

Table of Contents

Acknowledgments

This book would not have been possible without the assistance of many people. First and foremost, thank you to the patients, doctors, researchers, growers and activists who agreed to be interviewed and spoke with me at length, often revealing very personal information. I appreciate you sharing your stories in the hopes of changing the situation of medical marijuana. A special thank you to Amy Dawn Bourlon-Hilterbran, founder of American Medical Refugees, for welcoming me into the group and helping me connect with patients from around Colorado.

Thanks are also owed to the many friends and colleagues who gave advice on early chapters. Thanks to Priya Jha, Debbie Abbott, Kevan Brown, Mark Bunster, Carol Conzelman and Daniel Goldstein–I really appreciate your feedback. My appreciation to Amy Hayes for your expert help with graphs and images. Also, thank you to Leland Rucker for profiling my research and providing valuable contacts in the cannabis community.

Finally, thanks to my family. To my daughter, Lola, thank you for understanding when, for three years, I was always "busy on my book." To my husband, Tim Zych, I appreciate that you always believed in this project. Thank you for reading early drafts, giving feedback, and most importantly, urging me on even in my moments of doubt. I couldn't have done it without you.

Preface

I can clearly remember the first time I smoked marijuana. It was the summer before my senior year of high school. I was 16 years old. A friend and I had traveled to the beach with my family, and we had met some vacationing teenage boys. They were having a party at their hotel room one night and invited us over. One of the guys said he had a little bit of pot and asked me if I wanted to smoke some. Always open to new experiences and wanting to look "cool," I quickly agreed. The two of us walked from the hotel down to the beach; my friend stayed behind with the others. He also was in high school and didn't even have a smoking implement, so he made a pipe out of a Coke can. I have to admit that the experience was a bit of a letdown. I wasn't sure what I was doing, and the weed was pretty bad—I barely felt a buzz from it. But I wasn't turned off from trying it again, and I would continue to smoke sporadically throughout the rest of high school and college, eventually buying a pipe of my own and learning to tell the good weed from the bad.

However, it wasn't until I moved to Colorado in 1993 that I became more of what people would call a "stoner." I started dating someone who grew his own marijuana (still illegal at the time, of course) and began to smoke more regularly. My collection of smoking implements grew to include two bongs. I learned the difference between *indica* and *sativa* strains (the former is generally more sedating and the latter more uplifting), and I came to understand more about the plant in general. While marijuana was illegal in Colorado at that time, Boulder was definitely a stoner's town and the police generally looked the other way when it came to pot smoking. Most of the people I knew smoked weed, and I thought little about the fact that, as a successful teacher and PhD candidate, I did not fit the stereotype of the typical marijuana user. I would

1

continue to use marijuana after I graduated and got a job as a professor and after I settled down, got married, bought a house, and started a family. Eventually, I designed a course about the politics of drugs and learned more not just about marijuana but also about the drug war in general. I became an expert on the drug that had always been a normalized part of my adult life long before its legalization and destigmatization.

So why am I telling you the brief history of my marijuana use in a book about medical marijuana patients? Well, the fact is that despite knowing far more than the average American about cannabis,[1] I was nonetheless surprised when I started doing research for this book. I had long thought of marijuana as a relatively harmless drug. It might make you slightly sleepy or unmotivated or give you a bit of a smoker's cough, but it was nowhere near as dangerous as alcohol. Additionally, I was aware that it had some medical benefits—primarily pain relief. Still, I bought into a lot of the misconceptions around medical marijuana, believing that the medical movement was primarily a gateway to recreational legalization. I also thought that most medical patients were getting cards only to use the drug recreationally and that it certainly couldn't have all the "miracle" medical benefits that some proponents claimed. Despite years of use and research, I don't think I really took cannabis as a medicine all that seriously.

That all changed when I started hearing the firsthand stories of families who had moved to access medicinal marijuana. While it might be easy to discount a few anecdotal accounts, interviewee after interviewee regaled me with stories of near "miracle" cures. Sure, there were a few patients who did not have the hoped for response to cannabis, but not one of the dozens of people I interviewed recounted a negative reaction to the drug. Alternatively, I heard stories of children who went from near vegetative states to sitting up and talking. Kids confined to wheelchairs were suddenly able to walk. Patients whose organs were shutting down—who were on the verge of death—healed and went into remission. Veterans who had been completely incapacitated by post-traumatic stress disorder (PTSD) and anxiety were able to live almost normal lives. Others whose lives were hampered by chronic pain or depression or fatigue suddenly could reenter everyday life again. While each story seemed almost too good to be true, taken as a whole they could not be ignored. This drug is powerful, and more and more patients are discovering that power.

This book tells the story of some of the pioneers in the field of medical marijuana—doctors, growers, activists, and, most especially, patients. Because I am based in Colorado, my research primarily focuses on the cannabis community here, particularly those who have moved here to access the drug. Colorado is not the first or the largest state to legalize medical marijuana, but it has served as a beacon for many from throughout the country and world who are seeking better and alternative treatments in the form of the marijuana plant. In the chapters that follow I attempt to elucidate why that is, how Colorado came to be that place, and what others states could do or are doing to follow suit. Additionally I address the practicalities of medical marijuana uses, policy, research and whether or not moving to access marijuana is the right answer for patients. The politics around cannabis are uncertain and changing fast. Let this book be not only an archive of patients' stories but also a snapshot of a time and place and people that can serve as a template for those who follow.

The stories of medical marijuana refugees are central to this topic, and as such the book relies heavily on numerous personal interviews. When not otherwise cited, information in the text comes from my own interviews with those involved.

Introduction:
"Pikes Peak or Bust"

Pioneer: 2a: A person or group that originates or helps open up a new line of thought or activity or a new method or technical development; **b:** One of the first to settle in a territory.[1]
Refugee: One that flees; *especially*: a person who flees to a foreign country or power to escape danger or persecution.[2]

In January 1859 George A. Jackson, a miner with years of experience in California's goldfields, panned a half-ounce of gold from a remote section of Clear Creek in Colorado.[3] That same month, six men from a camp in Boulder Canyon discovered large quantities of gold at the foot of what would later become Gold Hill, Colorado.[4] At the time, there were few permanent settlements in Colorado apart from trading posts and forts. News spread fast about the discoveries, and soon newspapers in Kansas and farther east ran headlines such as "Pikes Peak, Gold Excitement in the City, a New California" (*Leavenworth (KS) Times*).[5] The entire eastern region of the U.S. was abuzz with talk of the new gold rush, and "Pikes Peak or Bust" became the catchphrase of the time. It is estimated that 100,000 new residents settled in the Colorado territory between 1859 and 1861, founding cities such as Denver and Boulder and creating boom mining towns like Central City.[6] Colorado's gold rush would forever change the territory, and the unprecedented numbers that settled in the region led to social, economic, and political transformations. Colorado Territory was formed in 1861, and in 1876 it became a state.[7] This early gold rush history would frame Colorado (and the west in general) as a repository of possibility for European Americans and set up the state for the thousands of people who would eventually move there.

Approximately 154 years after the gold rush, a new influx of immigrants began to flow into Colorado. These transplants weren't searching for gold, however, but rather a plant-based medicine to cure their ailments. Many of these new residents began to call themselves "medical marijuana refugees." While the term refugee has generally been reserved for those fleeing repressive international regimes of wars, the term was adopted by some of the early families who moved to Colorado for medical marijuana. It became part of the name "American Medical Refugees," a group that provide support to those who have to leave their state to seek medical treatment with marijuana without fear of legal repercussions. Although medical refugees might not be fleeing war in the traditional sense, they are fleeing the drug war. Parents who provide cannabis to sick children in states where it is not legal face jail time or having their children taken from them. Patients can and have died waiting for access to the medicine. They moved to Colorado because of its progressive marijuana laws, plentiful and varied medical cannabis supply, and welcoming medical and business community. As such, they became part of the latest chapter in Colorado history—not the "gold rush" but the "green rush." More than 200,000 people moved to Colorado in 2013 and 2014, immediately following the legalization of marijuana in the state by Ballot Amendment 64 in 2012.[8]

While there is certainly a plethora of reasons for the influx of new residents into Colorado at this time, including Colorado's strong economy and growing tech industry, legal marijuana definitely had a hand in spurring the migration. In fact, a survey by the Colorado Health Department estimated that up to four of five new residents considered legal marijuana as a positive factor in their move.[9] While medical marijuana had been legal in the state since 2000, recreational legalization undoubtedly increased the number of patients moving to Colorado to seek cannabis treatment. Not only did full legalization increase acceptance and availability of cannabis, but also Sanjay Gupta's 2013 CNN special, *Weed*, showed thousands of families the possible benefits of cannabis for their sick children. Many of these parents would decide to choose Colorado as their new home.

While Colorado is currently one of 46 states (in addition to the District of Columbia) with some form of legal medical marijuana, it nonetheless remains a favored locale for patients fleeing oppressive federal drug policy. Of the 46 states with some sort of legislation, only 33 actually allow patients access to the full marijuana plant. The other states allow only nonpsychoactive CBD-only oil (CBD, or cannabidiol, is one of over 100 compounds known as cannabinoids that are found in the cannabis plant and that will be discussed in more detail later in the book. CBD is not psychoactive like the better-known THC but does have various medicinal properties.).[10] Of those 33 states, most of them have legalized medical marijuana only in the last few years, subsequent to Washington state and Colorado's recreational legalization in 2013. Thus, for the start of the medical marijuana rush to Colorado, choices for relocation were much more limited. Even today many "legal" medical states do not provide for patients to grow their own medicine or are still working out licensing for dispensaries or grows, making the medicine nearly impossible to obtain legally. Americans for Safe Access, an organization whose mission is to ensure safe and legal access to marijuana for therapeutic use and research, has graded states on "patient rights and civil protection from discrimination, access to medicine, ease of navigation, functionality, as well as consumer safety and provider requirements."[11] Colorado comes in at a close second behind California, the first state to legalize medical marijuana in 1996. While many "refugees" have chosen to move to California, many prefer Colorado for its lower cost of living and the fact that it is closer to their home states. Additionally, Colorado has cultivated an extensive network of growers and researchers who are developing a vast array of strains and product with medicinal utility, often available at low or no cost. Finally, in large part because of the CNN *Weed* special's focus on the Figi family and the early CBD strain "Charlotte's Web," named for their daughter, many families decided to move to the Colorado Springs area, creating a network of medical marijuana patients and families who serve as a supportive community for newcomers. Much as international immigrants and refugees will often settle in the same area of a new country because of an existing network, medical marijuana refugees have done the same thing in the Colorado Springs area, giving new meaning to the nineteenth century catch phrase "Pikes Peak or Bust" (Pikes Peak is the 14,115-foot mountain that looms over Colorado Springs and the surrounding area).

While medical marijuana legalization and the concurrent boom in patients using the medicine are fairly recent phenomena in the United States, the reality is that cannabis has been used medicinally across the globe for thousands of years. "Ancient peoples during the Neolithic period found uses for virtually every part of the plant, which has been cultivated by humans since the dawn of agriculture more than 10,000 years ago."[12] In fact, recent archaeological findings show that cannabis has been used in China for both recreational and medical uses since long before the time of Christ. The first reference specifically to the medicinal use of marijuana dates to 2700 BC, in the *Pen Ts'ao Chen*, the pharmacopeia of Shen Nung, known as the "father of traditional Chinese medicine." Shen Nung recommended cannabis for over 100 ailments, and Chinese doctors often used marijuana as a painkiller for surgery.[13] Cannabis was also a part of traditional Hindu worship and Ayurvedic medicine in India. The plant is mentioned in ancient Vedic texts and was believed to promote "longevity and good health."[14] In addition to being a religious sacrament for Hindu holy men, often consumed as bhang (a cannabis-infused drink), marijuana is also recognized to have been used throughout history by Indian folk healers. Marijuana was known to healers as "ganja," and they used the medicinal plant for "relieving anxiety, lowering fevers, overcoming fatigue, enhancing appetite, improving sleep," and more.[15]

From China and India, cannabis found its way to Europe, where locals quickly learned of its medical uses. It was used by early Hebrew and Christian healers, and the second century Greek physician Galen noted its beneficial medical properties. The first illustration of the plant in Western literature appears in Dioscorides' *Materia Medica*, a Byzantine manuscript considered the "foundation for all modern pharmacopeias." Another European, Swedish botanist Carl Linnaeus, gave the plant its modern name, *Cannabis sativa*, in 1753. Before being brought to the Americas cannabis had been used medicinally for hundreds of years in Europe. Nicolas Culpeper's *Compleat Herbal* was published in mid–17th century England and would serve as the standard reference on medicinal plants for the next three hundred years. It recommended hemp (as cannabis was known in the region at the time) as a treatment for burns, gout, stomach problems, and general pain relief among other ailments. *The New London Dispensary*, published in 1682, also included cough and jaundice in the list of ailments that cannabis could benefit.[16]

Not only was "hemp" known as a folk herbal cure in pre-20th century Europe, the British also began the first modern medical studies of the drug in the 19th century. In 1848 Dr. William O'Shaughnessy, an Irish doctor serving with the British East India Company, published the results of a series of observational studies he conducted on "Indian Hemp" in Nepal, Persia, and Afghanistan. In his research, he gave oral cannabis extract to patients with "rabies, cholera, tetanus, epilepsy, rheumatism," and other hard-to-treat conditions. His groundbreaking research demonstrated that cannabis had many of the healing properties currently being rediscovered by 21st century patients, including "efficacy as a pain-killer, a muscle relaxant, and 'an anti-convulsant remedy of the greatest value.'" O'Shaughnessy returned to London with a stash of hemp that he gave to a local pharmacist, Peter Squire. The pharmacist created an alcohol-based tincture he called "Squire's Extract," which was prescribed for conditions such as nausea, delirium tremens, epilepsy, and spasms.[17]

Cannabis's medicinal properties were also being recognized across the Atlantic at the time. The 1854 U.S. Pharmacopeia listed Indian Hemp as a medicine, and by the end of the nineteenth century more than 100 articles had appeared in medical journals lauding the benefits of this "wonder drug."

In 1860 "the Ohio Medical Society conducted the first official U.S. government study of cannabis, surveying the medical literature and cataloguing an impressive array of conditions that doctors had successfully treated with psychoactive hemp."[18] These conditions ranged from bronchitis to postpartum depression to migraine headaches. In fact, it was not unusual at all for patients in late nineteenth century America to be prescribed some sort of cannabis product for their ailments. *The Antique Cannabis Book*, an online compendium of all known medicinal cannabis products prior to the drug's prohibition, lists more than 2,000 "tinctures, extracts, home brews, corn remedies, anti-asthmatic cigarettes, cough syrups, migraine headache products, veterinary medicines, prescription drugs, and other products."[19] Clearly, cannabis was a popular, widely used medicine until just under a century ago.

If cannabis has a long history of medicinal use throughout the world, including somewhat recently in the U.S., why is it still considered an alternative or experimental treatment? Why is it widely rejected by

THE

DISPENSATORY

OF THE

UNITED STATES OF AMERICA

BY

GEORGE B. WOOD, M.D.,

PRESIDENT OF THE AMERICAN PHILOSOPHICAL SOCIETY;
PRESIDENT OF THE COLLEGE OF PHYSICIANS OF PHILADELPHIA;
EMERITUS PROFESSOR OF THE THEORY AND PRACTICE OF MEDICINE IN THE UNIVERSITY
OF PENNSYLVANIA, ETC. ETC.,

AND

FRANKLIN BACHE, M.D.,

LATE PROFESSOR OF CHEMISTRY IN JEFFERSON MEDICAL COLLEGE OF PHILADELPHIA;
LATE VICE-PRESIDENT OF THE COLLEGE OF PHYSICIANS OF PHILADELPHIA;
LATE PRESIDENT OF THE AMERICAN PHILOSOPHICAL SOCIETY, ETC. ETC.

THIRTEENTH EDITION,
CAREFULLY REVISED.

PHILADELPHIA:
J. B. LIPPINCOTT AND CO.
1876.

Above and opposite page: The United States Pharmacopeia (USP) is a compendium of drug information that has been published annually since 1820 under the authorship of the nonprofit U.S. Pharmacopeial Convention. The USP establishes written and physical standards for medicines and is used by insurance companies to develop formularies. Cannabis was listed in various forms from 1851 to 1940. This is the 1876 listing (courtesy antiquecannabisbook.com).

EXTRACTUM CANNABIS. *U. S.*

Extract of Hemp.

An alcoholic extract of the dried tops of Cannabis sativa, var. *Indica. U. S.*
Off. Syn. EXTRACTUM CANNABIS INDICÆ. *Br.*
CANNABIS. *Sex. Syst.* Diœcia Pentandria. — *Nat. Ord.* Cannabinaceæ.
Gen. Ch. MALE. *Calyx* five-parted. *Stamens* five. FEMALE. *Calyx* one-leaved, rolled up. *Styles* two. *Lindley.*

Cannabis sativa. Linn. *Sp. Plant.* 1457; Griffith, *Med. Bot.* p. 572. Hemp is an annual plant, from four to eight feet or more in height, with an erect, branching, angular stem. The leaves are alternate or opposite, on long, lax footstalks, roughish, and digitate with linear-lanceolate, serrated segments. The stipules are subulate. The flowers are axillary; the male in long, branched, drooping racemes; the female in erect simple spikes. The stamens are five, with long pendulous anthers; the pistils two, with long, filiform, glandular stigmas. The fruit is ovate and one-seeded. The whole plant is covered with a fine pubescence, scarcely visible to the naked eye, and is somewhat viscid to the touch. The hemp plant of India, from which the drug is derived, has been considered by some as a distinct species, and named *Cannabis Indica;* but the most observant botanists, upon comparing it with our cultivated plant, have been unable to discover any specific difference. It is now, therefore, regarded merely as a variety, and is distinguished by the epithet *Indica.* Dr. Pereira states that, in the female plant, the flowers are somewhat more crowded than in the common hemp; but that the male plants in the two varieties are in all respects the same. It is unfortunate that the name of *Indian hemp* has been attached to the medicinal product; as, in the United States, the same name has long been appropriated to *Apocynum cannabinum;* and some confusion has hence arisen.

C. sativa is a native of the Caucasus, Persia, and the hilly regions in the north of India. It is cultivated in many parts of Europe and Asia, and largely in our Western States. It is from the Indian variety exclusively that the medicine is

the medical establishment? And why, in 2015, did the acting Drug Enforcement Administration (DEA) chief, Chuck Rosenberg, feel free to state, "What really bothers me is the notion that marijuana is also medicinal—because it's not.... [D]on't call it medicine—that is a joke."?[20] The answer to these questions is complicated but rests in large part on a racist propaganda campaign started by Harry J. Anslinger in the early 20th century. Anslinger's campaign would eventually lead to the prohibition of cannabis and its inclusion as a Schedule I drug in the Controlled Substances Act of 1971, a legal move that initiated the contemporary drug war on marijuana.

Anslinger, the son of European immigrants, was born in Pennsylvania in 1892.[21] He was not able to join the military because he was blind in one eye, so he spent his early career working for a variety of military and police organizations.[22] In 1929 his career took a turn, as he was appointed assistant commissioner in the United States Bureau of Prohibition. However, alcohol prohibition had been a huge failure, with

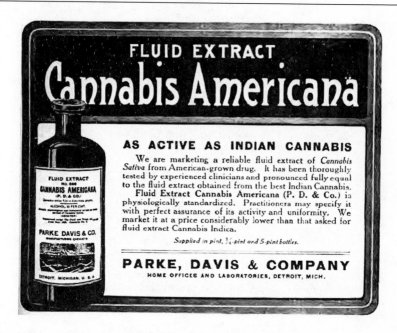

By the late 1800s, most pharmaceutical companies were producing and selling cannabis tinctures. Parke, Davis and Company (now owned by Pfizer) developed a potent indica strain called Cannabis Americana in 1896 (courtesy antiquecannabisbook.com).

crime and gang violence flourishing. There was also a growing public health crisis due to rising alcohol consumption and toxic products due to unregulated alcohol production. As Prohibition began to crumble (it would eventually be repealed with the 21st Amendment in 1933), the Treasury Department, which oversaw the Bureau of Prohibition, created a new agency, the Federal Bureau of Narcotics (FBN), and put Anslinger in charge, a position he would hold until 1962.[23] As Johann Hari writes in *Chasing the Scream*, Anslinger was immediately aware of the fragility of his new position: "A war on narcotics alone—cocaine and heroin, outlawed in 1914—wasn't enough. They were only used by a tiny minority." So Anslinger, who had previously described cannabis as a harmless drug, saying that it was "an absurd fallacy" that it made people violent, suddenly changed his tune. He realized that marijuana was the only drug with a large enough number of users to keep his department alive, and he set about to spend the rest of his life demonizing and fighting the drug.[24]

DRUG REPORTER   75

CANNABIS AMERICANA
U. S. P.
Physiologically Tested

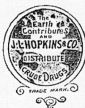

OUR American variety is the answer to the the question which has so long troubled manufacturers.

With our material a finished product can be turned out at a reasonable cost.

IT is no longer necessary to depend on the foreign variety which is of high cost and slightly superior. The uncertainty of further supplies of it is another factor favoring the American product.

J. L. HOPKINS & CO., 100 William St, **New York**

During World War I Americans had less access to foreign botanical medicines, including cannabis indica, imported from India. This ad from 1917 aims to convince consumers that American cannabis is also of high quality (courtesy antiquecannabisbook.com).

At the same time, William Randolph Hearst, the timber and media mogul, was concerned about the effect of hemp fiber on his timber empire. So he was an easy convert to the anti-cannabis side. He had long run anti-marijuana articles in his newspaper, so he was more than willing to increase the propaganda with patently false, racist stories involving marijuana. One such story would become the pivotal point in the public's opinion about cannabis. Victor Lacata was a 21-year-old Florida man who, according to neighbors, was a "sane, rather quiet man" until the day he smoked cannabis. The newspapers reported that the "marihuana" caused him to go insane and made him believe "he was being attacked by men who would cut off his arms, so he struck back, seizing an axe and hacking his mother, father, two brothers and sister to pieces." The fact that psychiatrists who later examined his file debunked this version of events, showing that he had long suffered from acute and chronic psychosis, mattered not to the thousands of Americans who were now convinced that cannabis could bring on insanity.[25]

It was also no coincidence that this story, focused upon by Anslinger and the media, was about a Latino. Anslinger was more than willing to use racism to his advantage in heightening the existing fear that the general population already had about marijuana. He tapped into deep-seated racial anxieties of the 1930s, since he knew that the two groups most feared by white America—Mexican immigrants and African Americans—were thought to use the drug more than whites. He claimed that the drug was especially pernicious in the hands of these two minorities and went so far as to state that marijuana made black men "forget the appropriate racial barriers—and unleashed their lust for white women." He even promoted the new name *marihuana* (the drug had previously been known in the U.S. as Indian Hemp) throughout the media to associate the drug with Mexicans, thus giving us the most common English term for the plant to this day.[26]

Despite the fact that Anslinger's campaign went against almost all scientific evidence (29 of the 30 scientists he contacted told him cannabis was not a dangerous drug), he soon realized that by controlling information about the drug he could control the public's perception—a key tactic in the drug war for the next 65 years. His campaign was crucial in bringing about passage of the Marijuana Tax Act of 1937, which essentially made it illegal to possess or sell the drug. As Martin A. Lee writes in *Smoke Signals*, "Yellow journalism, racial bias and political opportunism had triumphed over medical science." Anslinger's war on marijuana and scientific truth would rule U.S. drug policy until long after his death in 1975. By 1941 his propaganda campaign had resulted in the official removal of cannabis from the United States Pharmacopeia.[27]

This disregard for scientific evidence continued to influence drug policy throughout the fifties and sixties, and the drug war would find its next great warrior in the man who coined the phrase "war on drugs," the 37th president of the United States: Richard Nixon. Like Anslinger, Nixon saw fighting marijuana and other drugs as a way to fight what he considered to be "undesirable" members of society.[28] John Ehrlichman, counsel and Assistant to the President for Domestic Affairs under Nixon, said the following in an interview in *Harper's* magazine in 2016: "The Nixon campaign in 1968, and the Nixon White House after that, had two enemies: the antiwar left and black people. You understand what I'm saying? We knew we couldn't make it illegal to be either against the war or black, but by getting the public to associate the hippies with marijuana and blacks with heroin, and then criminalizing both heavily, we could disrupt those communities."[29] In support of his antidrug strategy, the Congress under Nixon ratified the Controlled Substance Act in 1970. This piece of legislation placed all drugs into five categories (or schedules) based on their safety, medical potential, and addictive qualities. Attorney General John Mitchell temporarily placed marijuana in Schedule I, the most restrictive category of drugs, pending review by a commission appointed by President Nixon. In 1972 the commission "unanimously recommended the decriminalization and possession and distribution of marijuana for personal use. Nixon ignored the report and rejected its recommendations."[30]

Marijuana's Schedule I designation not only flouted the commission's recommendation and thousands of years of medical use, it also made it nearly impossible for scientists to research medical efficacy of the substance. In addition, cannabis was now placed in the same category with LSD and heroin and scheduled as even more dangerous than cocaine and methamphetamine, which are Schedule II drugs. The Controlled Substances Act paved the way for increasingly harsh drug penalties in the 1980s and 1990s—set off by President Ronald Reagan's hardline policies and Nancy Reagan's "Just Say No" campaign. Reagan's administration marked the start of massive incarceration for drug offenses, leading to the U.S.'s now having over 2.3 million of its people in prison, the highest incarceration rate in the world.[31] The number of people in prison for nonviolent drug offenses increased from 50,000 in 1980 to over 400,000 by 1997. Today over half of federal prisoners are behind bars for violent and nonviolent drug offenses.[32] Although full medical marijuana (not just CBD-only) is currently legal in some form in 33 states and is fully legalized for adult use in 10 states and the District of Columbia, over 659,700 people were arrested for marijuana violations in 2017 alone.[33] And while the U.S. spends more than $51 billion a year on the drug war, it spends next to nothing on researching the medical benefits of cannabis, primarily due to the drug's Schedule I status.[34]

Thus, after less than 100 hundred years of marijuana prohibition and disinformation, we have lost access to considerable knowledge about cannabis as a valuable medicine while simultaneously arresting and prosecuting people for using the drug, whether for medical or recreational purposes. This brings us to today and the medical marijuana refugees in Colorado. Thousands of patients are choosing to flee government persecution in their home states in order to seek cannabis treatment for themselves or a loved one. And although California was the first state to legalize medical marijuana, and many other states now permit it, many of these self-declared refugees have chosen to relocate to Colorado in the last four to six years. The reasons for this choice are varied. Colorado was the first state to have high–CBD oil available for pediatric patients, and it still remains a leader in researching pediatric cannabis use and treating children with the drug. Additionally, Colorado's social atmosphere makes marijuana use more acceptable. With recreational legalization in 2013, more Coloradans than ever admit to using the drug, reflecting a more open-minded attitude toward it. This is in keeping with the western state's libertarian attitude toward personal freedoms as well as its residents' longstanding openness towards alternative lifestyles and medicine. Colorado remains at the forefront of alternative health and nutrition companies, with a wide variety of health-based companies and alternative healers such as rolfers and holistic and naturopathic doctors. These attitudes, of course, are not universal, and immigrant patients and families report many negative encounters as well as financial scams and outright robbery. Still, an overall welcoming attitude towards medicinal marijuana and cannabis patients plays into the decisions of many families and individuals to relocate to Colorado.

The state's policies also make it friendly to cannabis patients. The health care system allows parents to be licensed and registered as caretakers for their children, making it possible for them to stay home with their special needs children and receive a salary from the state for this important work. Many families who have moved to Colorado mentioned this provision as a key factor in choosing Colorado. Additionally, Colorado activists have been at the forefront of policy making for both recreational and medical users. Teri Robnett, a medical patient herself, has worked for over a decade ensuring that patients have the rights they need to easily access and use their medicine. This work has included fighting low limits on THC in the bloodstream for driving, opposing mandatory childproof containers for medical users (an issue because sick, disabled, and elderly patients are often not able to open these containers) and resisting other limitations on medical use. Other residents of the state have also become activists out of necessity, fighting for their own rights or those of their family members. Stacey Linn, the mother of Jack Splitt, found herself turned into an activist when her son was suspended from school after taking his cannabis oil with him. Linn proposed a bill that would require Colorado schools to let pediatric cannabis patients have their medicine administered at school. The bill passed and was signed into law by Governor Hickenlooper in June 2016. Although Jack Splitt has since passed away, the law now benefits all pediatric patients in Colorado who attend public schools, while students in many other states continue to face the same battle to access their medicine at school.[35]

In addition to having a strong tradition of cannabis patients' rights, Colorado is also at the U.S. forefront of medical research involving cannabis. There are currently hundreds of doctors who will recommend cannabis to patients in Colorado (651 physicians recommended marijuana for registered patients as of June 2017), and many MDs have extensive knowledge and experience working with medical marijuana patients, including pediatric patients.[36] Additionally, in 2015 the Colorado Department of Public Health and Environment awarded $9 million in grants for Colorado researchers to study medical marijuana.[37] These studies are being conducted at various Colorado hospitals on topics such as cannabis and PTSD, cannabis and pediatric epilepsy, and cannabis and palliative care for cancer patients. Due to the limitations on receiving federal funds for medical marijuana, these grants are a huge step forward for cannabis research in the U.S.

Because of the social, political, and medical benefits for cannabis users in Colorado, the state continues to attract patients from around the country and around the world. As with traditional refugee communities, once a group starts to settle into an area a community forms and more refugees tend to move to that area. In sociological theory, this concept is referred to as the "chain of migration"—migrants from a particular town or area follow others from that same community to a new location. They then form "ethnic enclaves" where they are able to keep personal networks, languages, foods, religions, and cultures alive.[38] For medical marijuana refugees in Colorado, that area has primarily been Colorado Springs due to its cheaper cost of living and proximity to hospitals and the health care

SOME POTENTIAL THERAPEUTIC USES OF CANNABIS

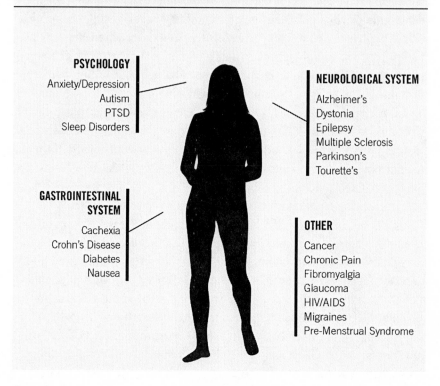

PSYCHOLOGY
Anxiety/Depression
Autism
PTSD
Sleep Disorders

NEUROLOGICAL SYSTEM
Alzheimer's
Dystonia
Epilepsy
Multiple Sclerosis
Parkinson's
Tourette's

GASTROINTESTINAL SYSTEM
Cachexia
Crohn's Disease
Diabetes
Nausea

OTHER
Cancer
Chronic Pain
Fibromyalgia
Glaucoma
HIV/AIDS
Migraines
Pre-Menstrual Syndrome

Some of the many medical issues that can be treated with cannabis (NORML.org).

available in Denver. This community has also been aided by the formation of the American Medical Refugees Foundation (AMRF) by Amy Dawn Bourlon-Hiltebran, who herself moved to Colorado to seek cannabis treatment for her son. Bourlon-Hiltebran's organization provides online resources for families and patients, as well as a variety of events throughout the year to help new Colorado residents find friends and community. AMRF also has liaisons with a variety of other medical cannabis groups, including Weed for Warriors, a group that advocates for another large refugee population—veterans seeking treatment for PTSD.

As the movement for access to medical marijuana begins to snowball throughout the United States and the world, Colorado stands to serve as a model for policy and research. By examining the stories of those who have fled to Colorado seeking treatment for themselves and their families—as well as the stories of those Coloradans who are developing and providing medical cannabis products, researching and recommending it to patients, and organizing and advocating in the community and government—this book will provide a template for medical marijuana regulation. Additionally, these stories and the concomitant information provided can serve as a guideline for patients who themselves may be considering a move to access medical cannabis. Finally, the hardships faced by Colorado's medical marijuana refugees, along with the research and experience we already have involving cannabis, prove that this drug must be de-scheduled on a federal level and made accessible to patients and families throughout the country. For the thousands of people suffering from intractable epilepsy, PTSD, cancer, Crohn's disease, autism, and more, time is not on their side. The federal government must act to legalize cannabis for medical use, and it must act now.

CHAPTER 1

What About the Children?

Tommy Turner sits on the roof of his Denver hotel in the darkness, stirring the mixture on his stove. He follows the directions on the YouTube video and hopes his first-ever batch of pot brownies will turn out okay. Meanwhile, his 14-year-old son, Coltyn, moves around the room spraying Febreze in the hope that the smell of marijuana will not waft into the hallway. They are both nervous about being caught. Tommy feels "guilty, sad, scared and hypocritical." When the brownies are done, Tommy cuts them into small pieces and tries a few himself to make sure they taste okay. They seem to have turned out fine, so he turns and feeds them to his teenaged son.

Turner could have never imagined his life taking this turn, but everything changed for his family three years earlier. Then, 11-year-old Coltyn was an average kid in rural Jerseyville, Illinois. However, that all changed one summer day at Boy Scout camp. The camp had a muddy lake with a floating dock in the middle that the boys loved to swim to. Coltyn had never been a particularly athletic kid; he was small and suffered from frequent stomach problems. He remembers getting tired that day as he tried to swim to the dock. About halfway across, Coltyn grabbed for a swim rope, hoping to take a rest. But the rope was not attached, and Coltyn sank under, gulping in mouthfuls of dirty lake water. The next thing he knew, he was being dragged from the lake, vomiting up muddy liquid. He had never lost consciousness, but he had taken in a lot of water.

The muddy Midwestern lake water led to an intestinal bacterial infection that had to be fought with antibiotics. For most kids, that would have been the end to a scary and unpleasant experience. But Coltyn had a latent case of Crohn's disease, and the bacterial infection activated it. The disease, which is a chronic inflammatory condition of the gastrointestinal tract that attacks both good and bad bacteria and begins to destroy the intestinal tract, affects upwards of 700,000 Americans. Named after Dr. Burrill B. Crohn, who first described it in 1932, the disease belongs to a group of disorders know as inflammatory bowel diseases (IBD). Symptoms include persistent diarrhea, abdominal cramps and pain, fever, loss of appetite, weight loss, fatigue, and, in children, delayed growth and development. The exact cause of the disease is unknown, but it has been found to have a genetic component.[1] In Coltyn's case, the infection from the lake water triggered his Crohn's, leading from occasional stomach problems to more and more severe symptoms of gastrointestinal distress. It all started with what seemed like a stomach flu that never went away. Then he developed worsening bouts of diarrhea, followed by weight loss and, eventually, weakness and fatigue.

The Turners spent the next three years fighting Coltyn's constantly worsening disease. They visited doctor after doctor, trying every type of drug to combat his chronic illness. When Coltyn tries to remember the lists of drugs, he gets confused because there were so many, He remembers only the side effects, which were oftentimes much worse than the disease itself. The first line of defense that western[2] medicine had to offer him was an anti-inflammatory drug called Asacol, which is an oral 5-amino salicylate. Coltyn describes it as essentially "stomach aspirin," and, as for most IBD sufferers, it did nothing to relieve his symptoms. Steroids are another common treatment for Crohn's, and Coltyn was started on prednisone, a corticosteroid. He quickly developed the common side effects of steroids, including red skin, a "moon" face, and brittle bones. He had to wear a cast on his foot for three months because his heel bone had deteriorated so badly. Fortunately, since he was still growing when the steroids were discontinued, his bone grew back, and the cast was removed.

Because Crohn's is a type of autoimmune disorder, immunosuppressant drugs are often a part of treatment, and Coltyn was no exception. He was tried on Rimicade, which led to rheumatoid arthritis and medically induced lupus. Next came Methotrexate, which gave him a 15-minute nosebleed after the first injection. Finally, he was put on Humira, a drug that was more effective than anything he had tried to date. He started to grow again, although he still suffered from such bad diarrhea that his parents had the bathroom in his house remodeled to include an outlet by the toilet so he could play video games while he spent time there. In his recollections of that time in his life, he spent

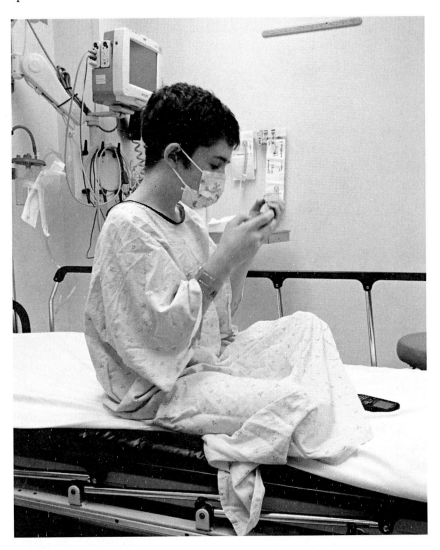

Above and following page: **Coltyn Turner spent huge amounts of time in the hospital after being diagnosed with Crohn's disease at the age of 11 and almost died before moving to Colorado to try cannabis for his condition (courtesy Wendy Turner).**

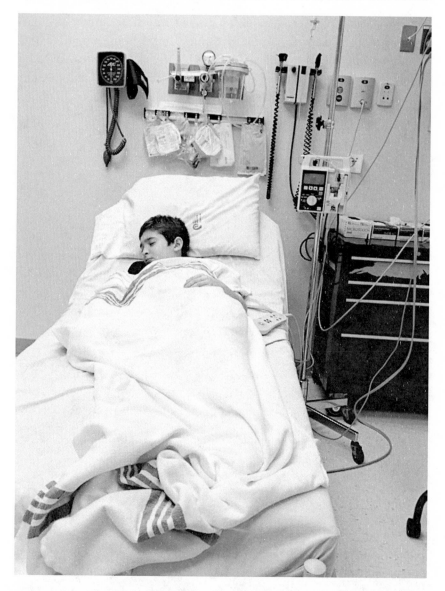

more time in the bathroom than not. And while the Humira was some-what effective its side effects were often worse than the disease itself. His lymph glands swelled up to the size of golf balls, and his doctors could not determine the cause. Their fear, though, was that he was developing a known side effect of immunosuppressant drugs—T cell lymphoma. He was immediately discontinued from his pharmaceuticals.

The swollen glands went away, but his Crohn's symptoms returned worse than ever. By the time he reached the end of his 13th year, he was confined to a wheelchair, was able to stand for only a minute at a time, and was suffering from constant pain and fatigue. He feared that his 14th birthday would be his last.

After the discontinuation of the Humira, the doctors gave the Turners three options for Coltyn's treatment. He could try yet another immunosuppressant pharmaceutical, with the concomitant risk of cancer (approximately a 66 percent chance of developing lymphoma), or he could try surgery to remove the damaged part of his colon. There was no guarantee that this procedure would work for Coltyn, considering that around 60 percent of those who have this surgery suffer a recurrence of symptoms within ten years. In addition, the surgery was counter-indicated for someone so young, since it would stunt his growth and he would have to carry a colostomy bag for the rest of his life. After delivering these two less-than-ideal options the doctor told the family that they could look into alternative therapies. The doctor legally could not state exactly what he was talking about, but he told them the words that would end up saving Coltyn's life: "Look into what is happening in Colorado."

What was happening in Colorado was medical marijuana, specifically cannabis oil. While marijuana had been legal for many years in several states, with California being the first to legalize medicinal use in 1996, Colorado had become a nucleus of medical use and research. Colorado legalized medical cannabis in 2000 with Amendment 20. However, it was a combination of the state being the first to legalize recreational marijuana in 2012 with Amendment 64, an overall open-minded stance toward marijuana growth and product development, and a state system that supported those with medical special needs that led to the state's status as an epicenter for the drug. When the Turners began researching cannabis oil, they came across the Realm of Caring, based in Colorado Springs, one of the first companies to begin manufacturing high cannabidiol (CBD) oils for medical use. With Coltyn's life at stake, Tommy reserved a hotel room, wrote down the Realm of Caring address, and drove his son to Colorado. Unfortunately, when they arrived at the Realm of Caring's address in Colorado Springs, it was simply a post office box. They did not know where to turn next. It takes time and residency to get a medical marijuana card (colloquially known as a red card) in Colorado, and Coltyn did not have that kind of time. So Tommy went to a recreational dispensary, where marijuana is available to anyone over the age of 21, bought a small bag of "flower,"[3] and went back to his hotel. And that is how a lifelong marijuana critic who had ended friendships over illicit (and what he considered to be harmful) marijuana use and had always told his kids "don't do drugs" found himself on the roof making marijuana brownies for his son.

Unfortunately, the marijuana brownies were not quite the miracle cure the Turners were hoping for. However, they did help enough that Coltyn continued to eat the brownies while they stayed at the hotel for the next five days. Tommy recalls that they began to get cabin fever in their hotel room, so they decided to take a drive into the mountains. At this point, Coltyn had been eating the pot brownies for a couple of days; they did not contain enough marijuana to make him "high," but he did feel a bit better. They stopped at a spot atop a ridge and walked about 300 feet to an overlook of the surrounding peaks. After taking in the view, Tommy started walking back to the car with Coltyn trailing behind. This was normal, because Tommy walks fast and Coltyn never had very much energy. Then, suddenly, Tommy was hit in the back with a snowball. He turned to see Coltyn laughing and running away. His first instinct was to make a snowball and return the attack, but then it struck him. This was a kid who could barely stand for more than a minute. Tommy hadn't seen Coltyn like this for years, since before the near drowning. It clicked. The marijuana was working.

Tommy immediately called Wendy, his wife, and they both cried at the news. They were still skeptical, but they could not deny that there was a change in Coltyn. Tommy and his son never went back to Illinois. They rented an apartment, got Coltyn a medical marijuana card, and found a caregiver with high CBD oil. Once Coltyn started taking medicinal oil at appropriate doses, his symptoms began to subside quickly. He no longer had to make frequent trips to the bathroom, his energy returned, and he began to catch up in growth. Six months after moving to Colorado and starting cannabis treatment, he went for a colonoscopy. It confirmed what they all suspected—Coltyn's Crohn's was in full remission.

Tommy rented a house in Colorado Springs. Wendy sold their house and most of their belongings in Illinois and moved Coltyn's brother, Skyler, sister, Ryleigh, and the family pet to Colorado. They became what hundreds of families have become in the past six years—medical marijuana refugees. Today the Turners have no regrets about the move. The family has settled in Colorado and made it their home, and the whole situation has led to a new vocation—political lobbying and testifying for cannabis patients' rights. Coltyn has become a spokesperson for the movement, and even wants to be a politician when he grows up. He is a normal, healthy 17-year-old kid, aside from one thing: he uses cannabis. Although he has finally found the medicine that works for him, with no side effects, cannabis's legally complicated status means that he has limitations. Unlike most 17 year olds, Coltyn does not even have a driver's permit, much less a license. He is too afraid of being pulled over and arrested for DUI. Because medical marijuana patients take the drug consistently, THC levels in their body remain high even though the patients' tolerance means they are not impaired. So driving is a risk. In addition, since marijuana is a Schedule I drug

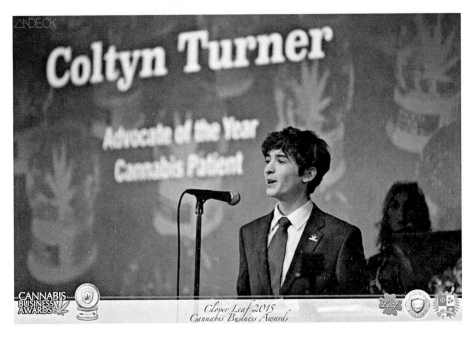

After cannabis put his Crohn's into remission, Coltyn Turner became an advocate for the medicine. Here he is shown receiving the 2015 Cannabis Patient Advocate of the Year Award at the Cannabis Business Awards (courtesy Wendy Turner).

according to the federal government, it is a felony to transport it over state lines. This means that Coltyn has been, in his own words, "a prisoner of the state of Colorado." He tried returning to Illinois once, without his cannabis oil, and he ended up back in the hospital with a flareup. It simply isn't worth it for him to try to cross state lines. So for now he and his family remain refugees in Colorado, using the medicine that works for him and continuing to fight for all Americans to have access to his lifesaving drug.

When the Turners moved to Colorado Springs in 2014, a mass migration of families seeking cannabis for their children had already begun. While Coltyn Turner may have been the first to try cannabis oil for Crohn's disease, children had already been using cannabis for seizure disorders for several years. Many families first learned about the effectiveness of cannabis for epilepsy through social media or word of mouth. However, it was Dr. Sanjay Gupta who first informed masses of people about the possibilities of cannabis, particularly for seizures.

On August 11, 2013, CNN aired Dr. Gupta's documentary *Weed*. This special was preceded by Gupta's article, "Why I Changed My Mind on Weed," in which he explained his change of opinion from his 2009 *Time* article, "Why I Would Vote No on Pot." In his new piece, the neurosurgeon and chief medical advisor for CNN explains how a year of research proved to him that marijuana did not deserve its Schedule I rating, not only because it has low potential for abuse but also because it has proven "legitimate medical applications." Dr. Gupta continues on to say, "We have been terribly and systematically misled for 70 years in the United States and I apologize for my own role in that." As Bruce Barcott notes in his 2015 book, *Weed the People*, one cannot underestimate the reach of a public statement of this sort from such a well-known medical professional. Barcott compares Gupta's statement to Walter Cronkite's repudiation of the Vietnam War, since Gupta had been such a proponent of the drug war for so long. Barcott states, "With the loss of Sanjay Gupta, the beginning of the end of the war on marijuana was upon us." In fact, as the CNN.com piece went viral, many Americans did have their eyes opened to a different side of marijuana, none more so than Americans suffering, or with family members suffering, from seizure disorders. One part of the documentary particularly grabbed the attention of those affected by epilepsy—the story of Charlotte Figi.

In 2013, at the time of the CNN special, Charlotte Figi was a six-year-old girl suffering from Dravet's syndrome—a severe form of epilepsy with onset in infancy. Children with Dravet's can suffer hundreds of seizures a day that generally do not respond to traditional pharmaceutical treatments. Due to the constant seizure activity, kids with this disorder often end up with developmental disabilities, and their lives are continually at risk since there is always a possibility that they will not wake up from a seizure.[4] Charlotte was no exception. She had her first seizure at three months old after a bath. At first, her parents thought it was a "fluke." After all, she was an otherwise healthy baby who was developmentally on par with her twin sister, Chase. However, as the months went by, her seizures became more frequent and more severe. Her family's lives were overtaken by frequent trips to the emergency room, where doctors performed every possible test. By age two her development had started to lag, and she was finally diagnosed with Dravet's. As with Coltyn Turner, the medical establishment tried everything it could to control Charlotte's seizures. She was tried on every anti-seizure drug, but as with most Dravet's patients these pharmaceuticals failed. Not only were the drugs ineffective at controlling Charlotte's seizures, but they also had terrible side effects. At one point, Charlotte's heart stopped after she was given a particular pharmaceutical, and she had to be revived with CPR.[5]

By the fall of 2011 five-year-old Charlotte was having 300 seizures a week and was catatonic, unable to talk or move. Her father, Matt, was serving in Afghanistan while her mother, Paige, tried to deal with Charlotte's seizures and also cared for their two other children. Matt, distressed at being so far away from his wife and family at such a critical time, decided to do what he could to help. He started researching Dravet's syndrome on the web and found a video of California resident Jason David treating his son's Dravet's seizures with cannabis. The videos showed the cannabis oil effectively stopping the seizures almost immediately. Back in Colorado, Charlotte's doctors were running out of options. They told the family that only two alternatives remained for her: putting her into a medically induced coma to stop the seizures or starting her on a powerful and experimental veterinary drug used to stop seizures in dogs. Her parents rejected these choices and decided to do the previously unthinkable: try marijuana for their child.[6]

While the Figis were lucky to be located in Colorado with its plethora of medical cannabis options, they were among the first in the state to consider using the drug legally for a child. Colorado's medical laws require that minors have two doctors' recommendations, but the Figis could not even get one doctor to consider the drug—until they met Dr. Alan Shackelford. Dr. Shackelford recalls that Charlotte had seizures on the way to his office, seizures in his waiting room, and seizures while he was examining her. Although he had doubts about recommending cannabis for a child, he was afraid that she didn't have long to live if she continued having uncontrolled seizures.

Once Shackelford gave his OK, another doctor followed suit. Soon enough, Paige bought a bag of a high–CBD strain of marijuana and with the help of a friend made an oil extract. When she started giving the oil to Charlotte, her daughter stopped having seizures immediately. Paige then started looking around the state to find a consistent source of high–CBD marijuana for her daughter. Several growers were working on these medical strains, but Paige met the Stanley brothers, who were already big players in Colorado's industry. Moved by Charlotte's story, they agreed to extract oil from their high–CBD plants for the little girl, naming the new extract "Charlotte's Web." They even agreed to sell it to the Figis for whatever the family could afford, an important consideration since medical cannabis is expensive and not covered by conventional insurance. After only one year of taking her eponymous oil, Charlotte's seizures were down from 300 a week to approximately one a week. As the number of her seizures reduced, her brain began to heal itself. After two years on a feeding tube, she started to eat on her own. She began to walk and talk and catch up in her overall development. Her story, as told in *Weed*, seemed like a miracle. The video of the once catatonic little girl now playing in the Colorado sunshine did more than touch the hearts of CNN's viewers; it provided knowledge and hope to thousands who were in similar situations.

By 2014 hundreds of families had moved to Colorado to seek out the Stanley brothers and their CBD oil. Many of these families had children with Dravet's syndrome or other forms of epilepsy, and, like the Figis, had exhausted the limits of conventional medical care. Contrary to popular belief, epilepsy is not a singular disease, but a family of disorders, often known collectively as "seizure disorders." There are currently around 3 million people in the United States with epilepsy of

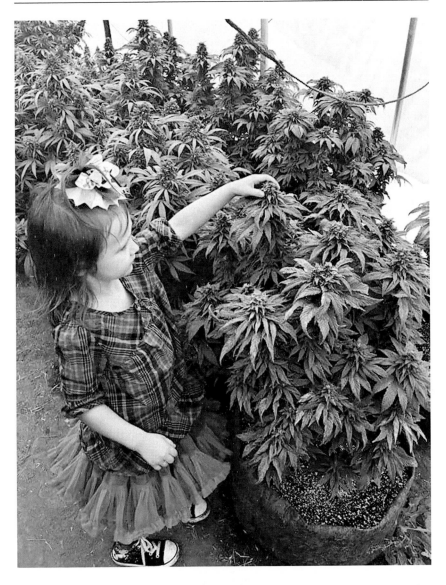

Pediatric patient Lily Pletka-Werth with the high-CBD strain of cannabis that saved her life (courtesy Vicki Pletka).

some sort, and about a third of those are not able to control their seizures with conventional medications. The standard definition of epilepsy is "a condition of the brain causing seizures, which are a disruption of the electrical communication between neurons."

There are multiple types of seizures involved in the various forms of epilepsy. Absence seizures are lapses of attention that last from around 10 to 30 seconds. They are most common in children and present as the child staring into space, sometimes with an accompanying movement like chewing or blinking. Sometimes called grand mal seizures, tonic clonic seizures are the type most people think of when they imagine epilepsy. Tonic clonic seizures start with loss of consciousness and a generalized stiffening of the body, followed by convulsive twitching. They generally last between one and three minutes and are considered an emergency if they last more than five minutes. Seizures can also be just clonic (all-over stiffening) or just tonic (twitching and convulsing), although these types of seizures are rarer. Atonic seizures, also known as drop attacks, involve an abrupt loss of muscle tone. They are most common in children, particularly those with a rare disorder known as Lennox Gastaut syndrome, and sometimes only the head will drop. Myoclonic seizures, the type most associated with Dravet's syndrome, are brief shock-like jerks of a muscle or group of muscles. Generally, the patient is awake and able to think clearly during the seizure. These are only four of the various kinds of seizures associated with epileptic disorders, complex conditions with a variety of causes. In fact, in 60 percent of cases the cause of the seizures is unknown. Such complexity and the fact that researchers are still discovering new forms of epilepsy and still trying to understand the complexity of the brain's neural system make seizures very difficult to treat, especially in children.[7]

Dravet's syndrome, the type of epilepsy Charlotte Figi and many of Colorado's pediatric cannabis patients have, is a rare and catastrophic seizure disorder that starts in infancy and is caused by a gene mutation that affects the way the ion channels in the brain function. Children experience frequent seizures, poor seizure control, and generally by the age of two have some sort of developmental delays that will persist. Of children with Dravet's, 85 percent have myoclonic seizures, although almost all types of seizures can be seen with this disorder. In addition, it is not uncommon for Dravet's patients to develop status epilectus, a life-threatening condition in which seizures last more than 30 minutes. Perhaps most frightening for parents is that children with Dravet's face a higher risk of SUDEP (sudden unexplained death in epilepsy), as well as other medical complications. Because kids with Dravet's often have multiple seizures every night, parents worry that each evening when they put their child to bed that child may not wake up in the morning.[8]

Unfortunately, despite the severity of Dravet's and other forms of pediatric epilepsy, conventional medicine has been largely ineffective at treating it. The roll call of pharmaceuticals used as anticonvulsants are not only often ineffective, but also have a long list of devastating side effects. The most common anticonvulsants used for pediatric patients are benzodiazepines such as clonazepam or diazepam (Valium), topiramate (Topamax), and valproic acid (Depakote). All of these medications are extremely potent drugs with psychoactive properties and potentially severe side effects, especially with long-term use. For example, the side effects of benzodiazepines include motor impairment, memory loss, confusion, psychomotor agitation, aggression, and irritability, and in long-term users depression and liver damage. These drugs are also highly addictive and lead to withdrawal symptoms that include anxiety, irritability, and more seizures.[9] Adverse events associated with Depakote, another form of valproic acid, include diarrhea, dizziness, hair loss, blurred vision, infection, chest pain, irregular heartbeat, swelling of the extremities, and loss of consciousness.[10] Despite the long lists of side effects and the fact that they are often ineffective, these medications continue to be the medical establishment's first line of defense against seizures in children as young as three months. It is no wonder then that parents have begun to look for safer, more effective alternative treatments for their children, including cannabis.

One such parent is Sue Root, who moved from Florida to Colorado with her daughter Amy in 2015. Sue had been struggling to control her daughter's seizures for four years, trying 15 different anti-seizure medications and seeing multiple neurologists with no success. At one point, one of Amy's doctor's told Sue, "Just take her home and enjoy her while you have her. There is nothing we can do." Sue is a registered nurse and is very knowledgeable about seizures and treatments, but she had never considered medical marijuana. In fact, she now states that she never "dreamed" she would one day give her child marijuana. However, in 2013 she saw CNN's *Weed* and started to change her thinking. She recalls, "I hadn't really even thought about medical marijuana and then I saw the Sanjay Gupta CNN series on weed and I started watching that and I was like 'wow that's really interesting.'" So Sue started doing more in-depth research on cannabis as a treatment for seizures and eventually decided to give it a try.

Amy Root's condition, however, is not as "simple" as that of some of the other children with disorders such as Dravet's. It all started on Sunday, January 24, 2010. It was a sunny late afternoon in Florida, and eight-year-old Amy was riding her scooter in front of her suburban house when she was struck by a car. She was airlifted to nearby Halifax Medical Center for emergency brain surgery. Although she survived the surgery, she entered a coma that was rated a three on the Glasgow Coma Scale—the most severe rating on the scale other than vegetative state and brain death. A rating of three essentially means that the coma patient has no response whatsoever.[11] After six weeks Amy opened her eyes, but her condition was still extremely critical. She was not expected to survive, but against all odds she did. Yet her traumatic brain injury meant that she was quadriplegic, unable to walk, talk, or eat on her own. She required round-the-clock medical care. Although she was severely disabled after the accident, Amy did not start having seizures immediately. She was on a multitude of medications at the time, including Kepra, a seizure prophylactic. At first her seizures were sporadic. However, within a year she had progressed to having full-blown, out-of-control grand mal seizures every day. In 2012 she was diagnosed with Lennox-Gastaut syndrome (LGS), brought on by her brain injury. LGS is a rare form of epilepsy accounting for only 2–5 percent of all childhood epilepsies. Children with LGS have multiple types of seizures that usually are not responsive to conventional anti-seizure medications.[12]

After the diagnosis, Sue, a single mother, struggled to find a way to control Amy's seizures. She was working as an RN, paying for full-time care for Amy, and making frequent trips to the hospital. Because of Amy's fragile condition, she would often suffer the rarest, most severe side effects of the drugs she was prescribed. Sue remembers a time when they went to the hospital and Amy was given the anti-seizure drug Depakote and then discharged. Within 24 hours of being home, Amy became completely unresponsive and had to be rushed back to the hospital. Her reaction to the Depakote was so severe (or "ferocious," as her mother puts it) that she remained hospitalized on a ventilator for three weeks. After so many pharmaceutical failures, her doctors recommended a Corpus Callosotomy (CC), a surgical procedure that severs the corpus callosum—the band that transmits messages from one hemisphere of the brain to the other. Amy had barely survived her previous surgeries, and although she was very disabled she was still responsive. Sue did not want to risk losing that. So she said "no" to the surgery, and when she later heard about medical marijuana as a possible treatment for seizures she was more than ready to consider it.

Always a medical professional, Sue Root researched marijuana and seizures for a year and a half before finally making the move to Colorado. She joined Facebook groups, talked to families using cannabis for their children's seizures, and consulted with medical professionals in Colorado. Like many other refugees, she had to explain her situation to family and friends who did not really understand why someone would move their child across the country to give them marijuana. In this case, that family included Amy's dad, since he and Sue were divorced. He would no longer be as close to any of his kids if they moved. Still, most people Sue knew, including Amy's doctors, supported her making the difficult move. Amy can't fly because of her medical status, so Sue, Amy, and her two other children drove cross-country. It took them six days to get to Colorado from Florida because Amy's condition means that she can't tolerate more than five or six hours of car travel a day. Fortunately, Sue does not regret her choice. Colorado's laws allow her to be paid to be Amy's nurse, meaning that she does not have to work outside the home as well as pay someone to look after her daughter, who needs constant care. Sue's adult daughter was also able to become registered as a CNA and receive a salary from the state to help care for Amy. Additionally, cannabis oil, while not a "miracle cure" for Amy, has improved her condition. Initially, like most seizure patients, the Roots tried high–CBD oil. However, Amy showed no improvements at all with that oil. In fact, many patients with LGS (and some other types of epilepsy) have not shown much improvement on CBD oil. So Sue tried a high–THC strain on Amy and soon saw an improvement in her seizures and her overall neuro status (more voluntary movement, for example). While previously Amy had 50–70 seizures a day, she is now down to 6–10 per day. Additionally, since starting THC oil, Amy's seizures are shorter in duration and not as severe. Now she rarely has a seizure lasting more than 10 minutes, whereas before she would have up to 20 thirty-minute seizures a day. While Sue admits that Amy's story is not one that includes

HEALTH EFFECTS OF MARIJUANA	THC	THC-A	THC-V	CBN	CBD	CBD-A	CBC	CBC-A	CBG	CBG-A	BENEFITS
Pain relief	■										Analgesia
Reduces inflammation		■			■		■		■	■	Anti-inflammatory
Suppresses appetite			■								Anorectic
Stimulates appetite	■										Appetite Stimulant
Reduces vomiting and nausea	■				■						Antiemetic
Reduces contractions of the small intestine					■						Intestinal antiprokinetic
Relieves anxiety					■						Anxiolytic
Tranquilizing/psychosis management					■						Antipsychotic
Reduces seizures and convulsions					■						Antiepileptic
Suppresses muscle spasms	■				■						Antispasmodic
Helps with sleep				■							Anti-insomnia
Reduces efficacy of immune system					■						Immunosuppressive
Reduces blood sugar levels			■		■						Anti-diabetic
Prevents nervous system degeneration					■						Neuroprotective
Treats psoriasis					■						Antipsoriatic
Reduces risk of artery blockage					■						Anti-ischemic
Kills or slows bacteria growth					■		■	■	■		Anti-bacterial
Treats fungal infection							■		■		Anti-fungal
Inhibits cell growth in tumors/cancer		■			■		■				Anti-proliferative
Promotes bone growth									■		Bone-stimulant

Of the more than 100 cannabinoids in marijuana, scientists know the medical uses of fewer than a dozen. This chart lays out some of the possible benefits of the various cannabinoids currently known (potguide.com).

a "miracle cure," she is very happy with the improvements she has seen with THC oil.

Although many patients, like Charlotte Figi, find CBD oil to be extremely effective at alleviating seizures, others, like Amy Root, do not get the results they had hoped from high–CBD cannabis. However, when they experiment with other strains of cannabis (whole-plant oils), some find that higher THC content helps their children. Unfortunately, a lack of research and understanding of the plant means that doctors are unsure of why the different cannabinoids work for some people and not for others.

What we do know is that cannabis contains 421 distinct compounds, at least 113 of which have been identified as cannabinoids. Cannabinoids are a group of chemical compounds produced by the cannabis plant that are primarily responsible for marijuana's effects on the human mind and body.[13]

THC (delta-9-tetrahydrocannabinol), marijuana's most well-known cannabinoid, was first isolated and synthesized by Israeli scientist Raphael Mechoulam in 1964. THC is most responsible for marijuana's psychoactive properties (its "high") but is also known to have many medicinal properties, including relief from pain, nausea, sleeplessness, and anxiety. Mechoulam and his team isolated the second most common cannabinoid, CBD (cannabidiol), around this same time. CBD is not psychoactive like THC, but it does offer many medical applications, including anti-inflammatory, anticonvulsant, antipsychotic, antioxidant, neuroprotective and immuno-modulatory effects.[14]

Cannabinoids were isolated in the 1960s, but it wasn't until the late 1980s that scientists discovered the receptors in the brain responsible for marijuana's effects. In 1988 the first receptors were discovered in the nerve synapses of the brain and were named CB1. The second group of receptors were found a few years later; CB2, as they were called, are primarily expressed in the cells of the immune system. The discovery of cannabinoid receptors helped doctors to understand how marijuana works to get humans high and also how it might have other effects on the mind and body. Essentially, when a person smokes or otherwise consumes marijuana, cannabinoids enter the body. As THC reaches the brain, it attaches to CB1 receptors and activates the endocannabinoid system. Thus, the user's reaction time slows, memory is affected, and judgment is impaired. Because CB1 receptors are located in the brain, the user begins to feel "high." Meanwhile, CBD enters the body and binds with CB2 receptors, causing a variety of physiological changes. Scientists are still researching the effects of the other 111 known cannabinoids on the brain and body.[15]

The discovery of CB1 and CB2 led scientists to hypothesize that the body must make its own compounds to bind to these receptors just as the cannabinoids from marijuana do. Again, it was Mechoulam and his team who identified, in 1992, the first of the body's own cannabinoids (coined endocannabinoids)—anandamide, which binds to CB1. A few years later a second endocannabinoid was discovered—2AG, which binds to the CB2 receptors.[16] The discovery of the endocannabinoid system and the understanding of its importance in the body's healthy functioning have opened up an entirely new area of medical research and also helped scientists to understand the role of cannabis in restoring balance to this newfound system.

While this is a very brief and simplified version of the history of cannabinoid research, it points to the complexity of cannabinoids and the endocannabinoid system. In addition to the 100+ known cannabinoids found in marijuana, there are hundreds of other compounds, including alkaloids, flavonoids, and terpenoids (essential aromatic oils). It is still unknown how each of the compounds affects the human body, but we do know that whole-plant cannabis has an entourage effect, in which the combined compounds multiply the effects of each individual cannabinoid.[17] This helps to explain why high–CBD strains of marijuana are effective at stopping certain patients' seizures, while other patients respond only to high–THC strains. It also explains why pharmaceutical forms of cannabis like Marinol (a synthetic form of THC used for its antiemetic effect) and Sativex, a cannabinoid medicine used for cancer pain and the treatment of spasticity associated with multiple sclerosis, are generally not as effective at relieving symptoms as whole-plant therapies (the phrase "whole-plant therapies" refers not just to the smoking or vaporizing of the leaf or flower but any use of extracts that come from the whole-plant, rather than individually synthesized cannabinoids). What most doctors, scientists, and patients can agree on is that more research is needed in order to understand how cannabis affects the mind and body and how to use the plant to its full medicinal benefit.

Unfortunately, our lack of knowledge of cannabinoids is not the only thing standing in the way of effective treatment for patients. Two major issues currently face the medical marijuana community: first, CBD-only laws, and second, the involvement of pharmaceutical companies. As many Colorado refugee stories attest, oftentimes high–CBD marijuana is not effective for children and other patients. Yet, because CBD is considered "nonpsychoactive," many states have begun to pass "CBD only" laws, allowing only medical marijuana that does not contain significant amounts of THC. In fact, of the 46 states that currently allow medical marijuana, 13 of those are CBD-only (and several, like Texas, are nonfunctional).[18] While many patients welcome any type of laws that will allow them to try cannabis, most experienced cannabis patients know that CBD-only laws are dangerous. By disallowing the beneficial effects of the whole-plant, these laws make states appear to be providing medical marijuana for those in need while also limiting usage to CBD-only oils and extracts. This means that patients cannot grow their own plants or try different types of whole-plant therapies.

These restrictions on patients' rights to use cannabis also benefit the pharmaceutical companies that are looking to patent and develop cannabinoid medicines. GW Pharmaceuticals is a British company that is currently leading the way in developing cannabis-based pharmaceuticals. Their website clearly states their aim: "Our vision … is to be the global leaders in prescription cannabinoid medicines, through the rapid cost-effective development of pharmaceutical products which address clear unmet needs." They are the makers of Sativex, a cannabinoid medicine that is used for the treatment of spasticity due to multiple sclerosis. It is also being researched as a treatment for cancer patients but is not yet available for that use. GW Pharma has partnered with pharmaceutical companies throughout the world and has launched Sativex in 15 countries, with approval in another twelve (although it is not approved in the United States). Additionally, GW Pharma developed a plant-based CBD-only medication, Epidiolex, which became the first FDA-approved marijuana-based pharmaceutical in 2018. The drug is approved for the treatment of seizure disorders including Dravet's syndrome and Lennox-Gastaut syndrome. With this FDA approval, "the flood gates could open for other companies in the cannabis space—and for GW Pharma itself."[19]

Although many Americans might see the approval of cannabinoid-based pharmaceuticals as good news, most families of pediatric patients are not as pleased. The cost of such medicine might be covered by insurance, but if it is not it will range from $2,500 to $5,000 a month, far more than cannabis oils at $100-$1000 a month.[20] Additionally, patients are worried that the development of these pharmaceuticals will hamper the medical marijuana movement, as states no longer need to allow for dispensaries or, more important, to allow patients to grow their own medicine. In addition, Epidiolex is not a whole-plant therapy, so it is unlikely to help patients like Amy Root who need the full range of cannabinoids found in the plant. In fact, many refugee families, already disappointed by conventional medicines, say they will not switch to a more expensive, possibly less effective pharmaceutical. As Allison Ray Benavides, whose son Robby uses Charlotte's Web oil for seizures, told the *New York Times*, "My kid's stable. I'm not touching it.... I don't need a double-blind placebo-controlled study to know something."[21] While she and other parents welcome the news of successful drug trials, they are concerned about losing their ability to continue to treat their children with multiple strains and forms of cannabis therapy.

Unfortunately, while many refugee families find remission or relief from different cannabis therapies, some children do not respond to cannabis at all or have only partial relief of symptoms. In June of 2014 Cara Domer and her husband Andy packed up their belongings and loaded their seven-year-old daughter, Olivia, Olivia's younger brother and sister, and their dogs into the car for the long move from North Carolina to Colorado. They had rented a house, but upon arriving in Colorado Springs Andy had to return to his job in North Carolina, where their previous house was still on the market. Like most other refugee families, the Comers did not take the decision to move lightly. They were out of options by the time they decided to sell their house, quit their jobs. and move away from friends and family. They simply did not know what else to do for their sick daughter.

Olivia Domer was a typical, healthy kid for the first four years of her life. However, in May of 2011, when she was 4½ years old, she had a tonic clonic seizure while taking a nap. She was rushed to a local hospital, where she was admitted and underwent a series of tests. Olivia was immediately started on an anti-seizure medication and sent home.

She had no more seizures for 15 months, and her family thought the first seizure had been a fluke. However, as soon as she went off her medication, she had another seizure and was diagnosed with epilepsy. Over the next two years she was tried on ten different anti-seizure medications and underwent a barrage of tests at Duke Medical Center and the Cleveland Clinic. None of the pharmaceuticals worked. Olivia not only continued to have breakthrough seizures, but they actually got worse. In addition, the medications had terrible side effects for her, including, as her mother explains, "major hyperactivity, difficulty concentrating, difficulty comprehending basic information or directions, intense agitation and aggression, socially inappropriate behavior, being extremely 'doped' up to the point of not being able to function at all, dizziness, increased seizures, headaches, vomiting, apathy, decreased appetite, and visual changes." By the time the Domers went to the Cleveland Clinic for a second opinion, they were running out of hope.

Unfortunately, after a two-week evaluation in Cleveland, the doctors determined that Olivia was not a good candidate for surgery and that there was nothing they could do but keep trying different combinations and doses of pharmaceuticals. Cara was not willing to continue to watch her daughter suffer the horrifying side effects of the drugs or stand by and do nothing while her daughter suffered seizure after seizure that could eventually lead to irreversible brain damage or worse. She had been researching CBD oil and seizures, and she decided to give it a go. The family put Olivia on the waiting list for Charlotte's Web (by this time, demand was far outpacing supply for the Stanley brothers) and they got ready to move.

Olivia started on Charlotte's Web in December 2014, and her mother had high hopes that CBD oil would finally be the medicine to alleviate Olivia's seizures. Sadly, although she had a temporary improvement in behavior (she was still taking Depakote at the time), CBD did not turn out to be the panacea they were hoping for. In addition, once they got to Colorado and started seeing new neurologists, Olivia was diagnosed with Electrical Status Epilepticus of Sleep (ESES). ESES is a rare form of epilepsy consisting of subclinical seizures during sleep, with a typical age of onset of 4–5 years old. It is characterized by an unusual EEG pattern of spikes and waves occurring in over 85 percent of a child's sleep cycle (Olivia's tests showed that she was having this pattern for over 95 percent of her sleep). This type of epilepsy is extremely rare, occurring in less than 1 percent of pediatric epilepsy patients. While daytime seizures can be present, the main symptoms are behavioral problems and regression in cognition. Mental problems can include ADHD, aggression, emotional lability, and even psychosis. Unfortunately, ESES is nearly impossible to treat effectively.[22] It does not generally respond to conventional anti-seizure medications, and it did not respond to the cannabis oil that Olivia was taking either. Her family has tried every treatment available, but for the last year her cognition and behavior has started to decline. As of this writing, her family is once again considering risky brain surgery in a last-ditch effort to stop her nighttime seizures and allow her brain to recover and develop.

While cannabis has seemed like a miracle drug to thousands of patients who have relocated to access it, it is clearly not a panacea. Olivia is only one of many patients for whom the drug does not work as they had hoped. This is partly because, like any medication, cannabis is not going to have the same effects for everyone. However, unlike pharmaceutical medications, there have not been enough specific studies on cannabis and its effects for a variety of ailments, including efficacy of different strains and doses. What this means is that most refugees, including parents of sick children, have become, in essence, the researchers for the drug. They talk to the few doctors working with cannabis in Colorado, but mostly they talk to each other and simply try out different doses and combinations with their children. As Olivia's mom, Cara, puts it when recalling her difficulties in deciding on the proper dosage of cannabis oil for Olivia, "Our kids are completely guinea pigs and their lives are in our hands. It is such a burden of responsibility to carry. I have been so nervous to decrease or increase her CW because I didn't want to put her in more danger." Even for those for whom cannabis does work, the decisions are difficult ones. When the oils fail to cure or alleviate symptoms for a child, these decisions can be devastating. Families who are able to do so often return to their home states. Because their children have usually exhausted all options, they may be facing the worst outcome when they return. Other families use all of their assets to move to Colorado; if cannabis fails to help their kids they have no choice but to stay in their new "home" and hope for a miracle.

Fortunately, cannabis helps the patients who come to seek it out more often than not. Dr. Shackelford, one of the foremost physicians treating patients with cannabis in Denver, says that the majority of his patients who use cannabis receive some sort of relief from the drug. Additionally, the history of medical cannabis shows that it can be effective for much more than just seizure disorders or Crohn's disease, and patients in the U.S. have started to take notice. While most of the first pediatric refugees came to Colorado to try to treat seizures (in large part because of Sanjay Gupta's report), more recently refugees have begun to arrive looking for treatment for other disorders. One of the most accepted uses for medical marijuana in the U.S. has long been cancer, and many families have relocated to Colorado to try medical marijuana for their child's leukemia. Cannabis is most commonly used to alleviate symptoms associated with cancer and its treatments. This use of marijuana for cancer is so mainstream that it has its own page on the NIH's National Institute of Cancer website. The site lists human and clinical studies that have proven the efficacy of cannabis for such common cancer treatment side effects as nausea, pain, anxiety, sleeplessness, and lack of appetite. In addition to these palliative effects, some cancer patients have noticed a reduction in tumor size or lack of growth of tumors after they or their child starts using cannabis. In fact, the NIH cites multiple preclinical and animal studies that have shown promise for cannabis as a tumor-shrinking agent. While there is still much more research that needs to be done, some parents are beginning to seek out cannabis for their children who suffer from cancer.

On April 2, 2019, Colorado recognized this potential when Governor Polis signed a bill to add autism to the state's list of qualifying conditions for medical marijuana. The bill, HB 1028, had been introduced and passed in the last two sessions of the Colorado General Assembly, but was vetoed both times by previous governor, John Hickenlooper.[23] Before this bill was passed, patients who were looking to try cannabis for this reason needed to have another qualifying condition to legally access medical weed. This was especially problematic for children, who of course have no access to the recreational market. Despite the positive changes in Colorado, marijuana remains out of reach for most patients with autism. Out of all of the states where medical marijuana is legal, only six consider autism a qualifying condition. Still, many parents are finding ways to treat kids with autism with THC and CBD, and the results are promising.

When Lori Ginn first moved to Colorado with her severely autistic son, William, she was at the end of her rope. Although William was nine years old, he did not talk much, did not answer or ask questions, or communicate in any way. He would not eat and had to be fed through a tube. As Lori remembers it, he was literally wasting away. Additionally, he had massive emotional problems; he was very unhappy and aggressive, hitting his mom and refusing to comply with simple requests. After a year on cannabis oil, however, Lori describes William as a "different kid." He now talks in sentences, repeats lines from his favorite movies, answers questions, and heartily eats many different types of food. His emotional state is also completely transformed. His mom describes him as an extremely happy kid who always has a smile on his face. While previously he couldn't go anywhere, he now goes to summer camps, museums, and a new school. His mom says that before the use of cannabis he couldn't even look at other kids, but he now plays happily with them, telling all about his good friends.

William was first diagnosed with autism when he was about 2½ years old and his family was living in Asheville, North Carolina. His preschool teachers noticed his unusual behavior at school, such as rocking back and forth and staring at the wall. He was also shaking periodically, so he was taken to Duke Medical Center, where he had an MRI. The tests revealed that in addition to a diagnosis of autism, he was having five different types of seizures and was seizing around 100 times a day. Doctors diagnosed him with Lennox-Gastaut Syndrome (LGS), the rare seizure disorder shared by many of the pediatric marijuana refugees. Apart from his autism, William's story is similar to most kids with LGS. His parents spent the next six years trying everything to get his seizures under control. Every two weeks they would make the four-hour drive to Duke Medical Center for tests and monitoring. In total, he spent about 16 weeks in the hospital during that six-year period. He was tried on combinations and varying doses of 12 different anti-seizure medications, but nothing really helped.

When he was five years old, surgeons implanted a Vagus Nerve Stimulation (VNS) device in an attempt to control his seizures. The

VNS device is sometimes referred to as a "pacemaker for the brain" and is an electrode placed under the skin on the chest wall, with a wire running to the vagus nerve in the neck. The vagus nerve is part of the autonomic nervous system, controlling involuntary bodily functions such as heart rate. It travels from the heart, through the neck, and to the lower part of the brain. In order to disrupt seizures, the VNS device is programmed to deliver stimulation to the brain through the vagus nerve. Patients (or parents) can also manually turn on the device when they feel a seizure coming on.[24] Unfortunately, as with many epileptic patients for whom medications are not effective, the VNS device did not stop William's seizures.

Not only did William's seizures continue after his implant, but he also began having 10–15 grand mal seizures every day. Grand mal seizures are the type of seizures that most people imagine when they think of epilepsy: generalized tonic clonic seizures with a loss of consciousness and violent muscle contractions. Because of the significant danger of injury from repeated drop seizures, it did not take long for William's doctors to suggest what is generally considered the last resort for epilepsy patients—brain surgery. In July of 2013, when William was seven years old, he had the surgery that had been recommended for accident victim Amy Root—Corpus Callosotomy (CC). In CC surgery, the corpus callosum, a band of tissue that connects and transmits messages from one side of the brain to the other is cut. This disrupts the seizure impulses between the brain hemispheres. Fortunately for William, the Corpus Callosotomy did stop his grand mal seizures, but, as is often the case, his partial seizures continued daily.

While the brain surgery was only a partial success, a coincidence at the Duke Medical Center would lead to Lori's eventual decision to try cannabis oil for William and their subsequent move to Colorado. While at the hospital, Lori met Liz Gorman, who was there for her own child's surgery. Liz's daughter is the same age as Lori's son, also has Lennox-Gastaut syndrome, went to the same neurologists, and was having surgery the day after William. Lori and Liz became friends and stayed in touch over the next few years. Lori learned that the CC surgery was not effective for Liz's daughter and that they had decided to move to Colorado to try cannabis after her grand mal seizures reappeared. The seed was planted in Lori's brain, and when William's partial seizures continued unabated, she began to consider cannabis. At the time, William's autism symptoms were also worsening. He was refusing to eat and had to be fed through a tube, and the lack of nutrition was exacerbating his already severe medical conditions. Knowing about marijuana's appetite stimulant properties, Lori decided to take the leap and give William CBD oil.

At first, Lori made her own oil with flower that she bought locally or she had friends in "legal" states ship her tinctures. She knew that what she was doing was illegal, but she was willing to do anything to help her sick little boy. Even though she wasn't fully sure of how to make the oil and wasn't able to procure a variety of quality medicine for her son, William slowly started to make progress. His aggression and mood were the first to improve, and his appetite picked up shortly thereafter. Meanwhile, Lori's marriage had broken up and life in North Carolina was becoming more difficult. She felt little support from William's school or community, and few people understood what she was doing. She recalls, "I had been in Asheville for 15 years, and I had friends who just walked away. They couldn't take it. I was consumed with autism and epilepsy and I had no support. I had to go."

So in July of 2015 she sold her house and moved to Colorado with William. They quickly found a home in a canyon near a mountain stream. She found a job doing accounting, and William was able to begin at a local elementary school. Still, the first few months were hard. Lori knew no one, and the move was tough on William. Change is difficult for autistic children, and Lori at first doubted her decision. Was it worth putting William through this huge move on the chance of further improvement? She questioned herself every day. Fortunately, like many other families, Lori found support with the local cannabis community: business owners, growers, and other refugee families. In Colorado she received support and information that was completely unavailable in North Carolina. Dispensary owners and growers recommended strains and helped her with dosing. She contacted the Colorado Springs-based group American Medical Refugees and was able to meet other parents going through the same ordeal she was. They gave her advice and provided much-needed support.

Although it happened slowly, Lori and William made it through those first few months, and Lori started to see improvement in her son.

However, the improvement was not what she expected. His seizures continued, but his autism symptoms became less and less severe. While these results were a surprise for Lori, they were certainly a welcome one. Although she had heard of cannabis oil being used to treat seizures (and certain other disorders), she had not previously heard that cannabis could be a treatment for autism. Little did she know that she was at the forefront of one of the newest cannabis therapies. In fact, other than a handful of personal stories where cannabis has successfully treated autism, there is little known about the drug's effect on the disorder. Just recently, scientists and physicians have begun to take notice of these anecdotes. As Dr. Daniele Piomelli, a top neuroscientist and endo-cannabinoid researcher from the University of California, Irvine, notes, "An anecdote is a pointer. It's something that suggests something needs to be either proven or disproven." One of the first researchers to explore this connection is Dr. Giovanni Martinez, a clinical psychologist in Puerto Rico who is treating autistic children with CBD oil and recording the results. His findings so far have been positive and have echoed parents' stories. Additionally, a 2013 study found promise for the treatment of childhood autism with CB2, and more recently the Autism Research Institute has stated that cannabis has shown potential to treat autism symptoms such as "anxiety, aggression, panic disorder, generalized rage, tantrums, property destruction, and self-injurious behavior."[25]

Still, these studies are few and far between, and parents like Lori Ginn are left on their own, forced to move out of state to get treatment and to use their kids as "guinea pigs" to find the right strains and doses. They rely on one another and the Internet to gain the information they need to successfully treat their children since the medical establishment can't give them any answers or guidance. While the DEA loosened the regulations on marijuana research at universities in mid-2016,[26] for these parents it was too little too late. And the families who make it to Colorado are the lucky ones. Many parents are unable to move to get the medication their children need or they can't make it to Colorado in time to try cannabis and attempt to save their children's lives.

Heather Berry is one of those parents. In 2010 Heather was living her dream life near South Bend, Indiana. She and her husband had just had their second child, a healthy and happy little boy. Tanner was beloved by his older brother, and Heather's husband was thrilled to have two sons he would one day be able to wrestle and play sports with. This dream life did not last long, however. At just two months old, Tanner had his first seizure. It was only 60 seconds long and only in one arm, but his mother immediately became worried. At four months Tanner had a second seizure that lasted for 20 minutes. Local doctors immediately referred the family to a neurologist in Chicago. At this point, Tanner continued to develop normally, but he also had 13 more seizures before he was able to get the genetic testing that confirmed a Dravet's diagnosis.

The Berrys' next few years were similar to those of the many other families who have small children with Dravet's syndrome. Tanner was in and out of ICU and EMU, on and off of various medications, and undergoing therapy to restore skills lost from multiple prolonged seizures. At the end of his second year, he had three seizures that lasted more than three hours each. He had to be repeatedly intubated and suffered a severe injury. Despite multiple inhaled drugs and IV steroids, he ended up with an emergency tracheotomy and spent a month in the ICU. After his tracheotomy, he could no longer speak and had to communicate by clicking his tongue and pointing. Eventually he learned sign language. He also had to relearn to walk three times due to having a catheter drilled into the long bone of his leg to deliver emergency meds during his seizures. During all of this, Tanner's parents worked full time (Heather as a nurse, her husband as an active duty Marine) and worked tirelessly to get him the best healthcare available.

Tanner, like his parents, was a fighter, and by the time he was three years old he was considered high functioning for a child with Dravet's syndrome. His mom recalls, "He ran and climbed like a little boy should…. We had been told not to expect very much … [but] he overcame so many obstacles and just kept smiling." Nevertheless, Heather was concerned about the side effects from Tanner's medications. He was on three different anti-epileptic drugs at the highest dose recommended for his age and size. She had a friend in Colorado who was one of the first to use cannabis for a child and had seen the positive results. So she began to consider a move to Colorado. Then, one Friday in August, Heather and her husband watched the first episode of Sanjay Gupta's *Weed*. Like dozens of other families, seeing the results on that show convinced them to make the move and try cannabis for Tanner. Heather decided that she would move with the two boys sometime before Halloween, giving the family two months to work out the logistics. Her husband would have to stay behind because of his commitment to the Marine Corps. Two days later, on the night of Sunday the 19th, Heather was at work when she received a call from her husband that Tanner was seizing. Like so many times before, he was rushed to the hospital when his rescue medications failed to halt the seizure. However, this time the hospital was not able to stop the seizure either, and Tanner never regained consciousness. Tanner Berry had his fatal seizure just 48 hours after his family made the decision to move. They simply ran out of time.

If Tanner had been able to try cannabis, would he still be alive? Would he, like the dozens of other pediatric epilepsy patients in Colorado, have found a vastly improved life with cannabis oil treatment? And how many other children across the country like Tanner never get to try a medicine that could save their lives? When Heather Berry discusses this most painful chapter of her life, one thought stands out: "I wanted to at least try to ease the burden on his tiny body. I never got the chance. I never even had the opportunity to try, and I think that is so incredibly unfair." Despite the fact that cannabis has been used for seizures and other medical conditions for thousands of years and despite the fact that there are multiple studies and a multitude of accounts of its efficacy in treating epilepsy, autism, cancer, and other disorders, the federal government refuses to admit that the drug has medicinal properties. Meanwhile, after almost 100 years of information and research suppression, families don't have time to wait for the government and the scientific community to catch up. For thousands of children, time is running out.

CHAPTER 2

Inadvertent Activists

Back at the turn of the millennium, young stay-at-home mom Jennie Stormes could have never imagined that she would one day be an activist standing up to governors and introducing and promoting important legislation. In 2000 she had just left her job as a medical facility office manager to stay at home with her three-year-old daughter, Sidnee, and newborn son, Jackson. However, like many of the parents of pediatric cannabis users, Jennie's life changed suddenly in October of that year when four-month-old Jackson had his first seizure. While over half of infants who have a seizure will never have another,[1] Jackson ended up as one of the unlucky ones, having a second seizure a month later.

Like most children with seizure disorders, Jackson and his family would spend his early years trying to bring his seizures under control. He would not be diagnosed with Dravet's syndrome for another nine years, during which time doctors would treat him with surgeries, pharmaceuticals, diets, and more. As is the case with most Dravet's patients, these treatments would not only be largely unsuccessful but would also begin to take a toll on Jackson's health. By 2010 Jennie Stormes was a single mom, and she had moved from California to New Jersey to seek better education for her children (particularly Jackson, with his special needs). She had just started nursing school when Jackson got the diagnosis of Dravet's syndrome. More specifically, doctors said that he had "idiopathic, carthogenic, medically refractive epilepsy." In other words, they had no idea how to stop his seizures. By this time he had failed over 50 combinations of drugs (23 drugs in 50+ combos). He had also had two brain surgeries to try to stop his seizures—a right frontal lobectomy and a 2/3 anterior Corpus Callosotomy. Doctors had implanted a total of four Vagus Nerve Stimulators, all of which had failed. Finally, he had been tried on a strict ketogenic diet three times for a total of almost five years, but this special diet also stopped working (the ketogenic diet stresses foods that are low in carbs and high in fat and has been used in the treatment of diabetes, cancer, epilepsy, and Alzheimer's disease).[2] By 2012 he was making two to six med-flights a month from the family's home in rural western New Jersey, on the border with Pennsylvania, to a specialist hospital on the New Jersey/New York border. At this point, Jackson was on seven prescription drugs: Depakote, Kepra, Vanzil, Phenobarbital, Klonopin, Banzel, and Stiripentol. The lists of side effects from these drugs were long and included "blindness, kidney failure, liver failure and death." Additionally, Jackson was suffering from various mental effects from the pharmaceuticals, including suicidal ideation. Eventually, his doctor said, "He's out of options. He's gonna die."

Jennie Stormes had become a nurse in 2011, and with her newfound medical knowledge she had become more and more concerned about both the lack of efficacy of Jackson's prescriptions and their dangerous

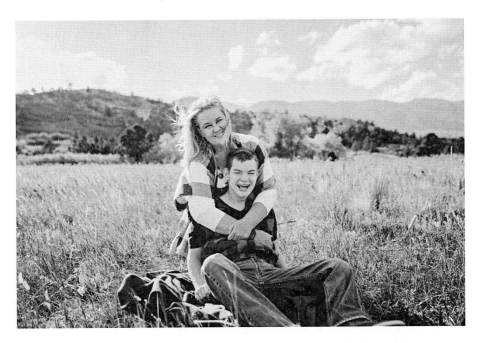

Jackson Stormes and his mom, Jennie Stormes, are able to enjoy Colorado's outdoors now that cannabis oil controls the seizures caused by his Dravet's syndrome (courtesy rachelcasephotography).

side effects. She recalls a doctor telling her of an experimental drug that Jackson could try. The doctor said, "I know of two kids who have tried it; one had seizure control and the other one died." Odds of 50 percent were not good enough for Jennie. In 2012 she attended a Dravet's conference and learned about parents using cannabis for their kids' seizures. At first she was skeptical, having always been taught that marijuana was a dangerous drug. But she was also aware of how risky the pharmaceuticals were, so she started doing research. She joined an online group and talked to parents from around the country who were using cannabis. Eventually she decided that there was "nothing to lose, and everything to gain," and she resolved to try cannabis for Jackson.

Unfortunately, while medical marijuana was legal in New Jersey at the time, the law was, as Jennie notes, "not set up to function for anyone, but especially not for children." In order for a pediatric patient to use the drug, parents needed to find three doctors to sign off for a card, a cost of at least $1,000 since these practices would not take insurance. Additionally, patients had to see a doctor every three months to keep their cards valid and were allowed to purchase cannabis only from one of the two dispensaries open in the state at the time. The cannabis that was available was selling for a very expensive $500 an ounce and was not of very good quality. The final blow was that patients could only smoke the medicine; oils and edibles were not available, but a special needs child like Jackson couldn't possibly be expected to smoke a joint.

So Jennie decided to take a big risk and try Jackson on cannabis without a card. Meanwhile, she became an activist. Because the situation was so difficult for patients in New Jersey at the time, Jennie joined with about 20–30 other families to fight for their children's right to cannabis medicine. Every week, on Thursdays, some of the parents would hold an educational protest in front of the Trenton statehouse, forcing the governor to walk past their demonstration multiple times. While many parents were not very vocal or loud in their activism, Jennie certainly was. Parents had shown up and protested at multiple town hall meetings with Governor Chris Christie with little result. When asked by parents, "What about our children?" the governor actually accused parents of wanting access to marijuana only so they could "get high." Finally, at a fifth town hall meeting, Jennie Stormes had seen enough. She confronted the governor and engaged in a lengthy debate about patients' rights in

New Jersey. Media reported it: "At a recent town hall forum, New Jersey Governor Chris Christie faced off with a registered nurse and mother of a 14-year-old medical marijuana patient about the state's failed medical marijuana program, and ultimately reluctantly agreed to consider changes to the law."[3] This would not be the last time Jennie would directly take on the government to fight for the rights of her son and other cannabis patients.

Meanwhile, Stormes' experiment with using cannabis oil for Jackson was going extremely well. Within weeks, the 14-year-old, who previously could not sit still for five minutes, could now watch one-hour movies at school. He went from being able to speak only about three words in total to being able to speak five-word phrases. Earlier, Jennie had been trying to wean Jackson off phenobarbital with no success (due to extreme side effects). Yet, within three months of starting cannabis oil, he was completely weaned off the powerful pharmaceutical. His mom noticed that many of the negative behaviors he had been exhibiting were not from his Dravet's but were side effects of the benzos. Once he was weaned, those behaviors went away. Yet, despite these successes, Jennie Stormes was concerned. After all, what she was doing was illegal in New Jersey. And because of her high-profile political activism on behalf of patients' rights, she became afraid of losing her child or at the very least being denied services. So in 2014 Jennie decided to move her son to Colorado, where they would be able to legally access the best forms of cannabis treatment for Jackson.

Due to the long history of activism in Colorado around marijuana and patients' rights, access to medicine was much easier for Jennie and for the hundreds of patients relocating to Colorado around that time. Because Colorado allows family members to become paid and certified caregivers for special needs children, Jennie and her daughter Sidnee, both nurses, were able to become Jackson's caregivers and receive salaries from the state. With the ability to stay home with her son and also have access to a wide variety of cannabis medicines, Stormes settled into what she hoped would be a quiet new life, outside of the political limelight. However, her new life as a stay-at-home mom and caregiver was not to last long.

In May of 2015 Jackson Stormes was suspended from Sand Creek High School in Colorado Springs after school officials found cannabis edibles in his lunchbox. As his mother explains, Jackson, then 16, was not capable of making the decision to take cannabis to school. With an IQ of 31, Jackson is not able to make his own lunch. Jennie had just accidentally packed the wrong lunch for him that day. Nevertheless, Jackson was suspended for one day, missing important therapy he received in school. And Jennie Stormes was once again thrown into the middle of a political fight—a battle that was already being waged in Colorado to allow pediatric cannabis patients to get doses of their medication at school.

This fight had been going on in the state for a year, led by Stacey Linn on behalf of her teenaged son Jack. In February of 2015, 14-year-old Jack, much like Jackson a year later, was suspended from his middle school in Jefferson County, Colorado, when school officials discovered that he was wearing a cannabis oil patch and that his personal nurse, who accompanied him at all times, was also carrying cannabis oil. Unlike in Jackson's case, Jack Splitt was completely aware of what he was doing. Jack was born with severe cerebral palsy and his mother had struggled with treating the illness since Jack was an infant. Before trying cannabis Jack was taking a variety of strong and sedating pharmaceuticals, many of which were used just to treat the debilitating side effects of the other drugs. Jack and Stacey lived in Colorado, so it was an easy choice for Stacey to try cannabis once she learned about the beneficial effects for other patients. The pictures of Jack before and after cannabis treatment tell the story better than words can. In the "before" pictures, he slumps in his wheelchair, mouth hanging open, eyes drooping, clearly heavily drugged. In the "after" pictures, he is alert and laughing, eyes smiling for the camera. His mother acknowledges that cannabis changed his life.

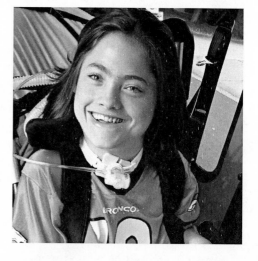

Jack Splitt used cannabis to control his cerebral palsy. This picture was taken around 2015, when he was suspended for wearing a cannabis patch to school (courtesy Stacey Linn).

Although he was still in a wheelchair, with constant nursing care and suffering from severe tremors and dystonia, the CBD oil improved his quality of life noticeably, reducing his life-threatening muscle spasms and allowing him to be weaned off some of the extremely sedating pharmaceuticals that turned him into a "zombie."[4]

So when Jack Splitt went to school with a CBD patch on and with his nurse carrying his cannabis oil, he really had no choice but to do so. He loved education; school meant everything to him. But without his medicine he could not attend school and participate in learning. Stacey thought that because medical marijuana was legal in the state, Jack had a red card, and he had only nonpsychoactive CBD oil he would be fine. However, school officials saw it differently. Sure, students could have highly addictive narcotics at school, but those were legal under federal law. In essence, the school officials were afraid of losing federal funding if they allowed any form of Schedule I marijuana on school grounds. Kathleen Sullivan, chief counsel for the Colorado Association of School Board Executives, told Aspen Public Radio, "There is no way around the fact that federal law still recognizes marijuana as a controlled substance under Schedule I. Our local boards are afraid to gamble on that federal money without reassurances that they will be protected."[5]

Despite resistance from the school board, Stacey Linn knew she could not send her son to school without his medicine, and homeschooling was never an option. Since she had years of experience with advocating for special needs kids, she immediately jumped into action. She founded the CannAbility Foundation to "provide support, resources, education and access to cannabis for parents of kids living with an illness or disability."[6] Soon afterwards, she worked with state representative Jon Singer to add an amendment to a marijuana bill being introduced in the state legislature. The amendment, known as Jack's Amendment, would allow caregivers to administer cannabis medications to children at school. Governor Hickenlooper signed the amendment into law in May 2015. Unfortunately, while the law allowed students to receive their cannabis medication on school grounds, it did not *require* schools to let students have access to their medicine.[7] That decision was still left up to individual school districts, and none of Colorado's 179 school districts created a policy around student access to cannabis, essentially meaning that the substance was still banned on campuses.

So the following year Stacey and Representative Johnson introduced a new bill, House Bill 1373, or Jack's Law, which would require schools to create a policy designating a location on school grounds where children could receive their cannabis medicine. If schools did not create guidelines, the fallback policy would be that students could be administered cannabis anywhere on school grounds by a parent or caregiver. When Representative Johnson introduced the new bill he tried to make

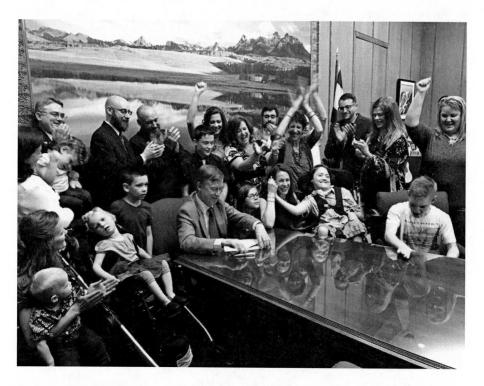

Cannabis advocates and patients witness Governor John Hickenlooper signing House Bill 373, or Jack's Law, requiring schools to allow pediatric medical patients to have their cannabis medicine administered on school grounds. Pictured from left, sitting at table: Rachael Selmeski, holding her son Maddox Selmeski, her daughter Maggie Selmeski, in stroller, Governor John Hickenlooper, Cooper Splitt, Stacey Linn, her son Jack Splitt, in wheelchair, Jackson Stormes. From left, standing: Meagan Patrick, holding daughter Addy Patrick (son Colin Patrick standing to the front), Senator Chris Holbert, Representative Jonathan Singer, Brad Wann, Benjamin Wann, Amber Wann, Amy Dawn Bourlon-Hilterbran, Jordan Wellington, Teri Robnett, Josh Kappel, Judy Linn, Jackson's mother Jennie Stormes.

it clear that not receiving their medicine was not an option for the nearly 400 children in Colorado taking cannabis, so it should not be an option for schools to prohibit their getting the medication at school. Doing so was essentially preventing these children from getting an education. To back him up, dozens of families with children who used cannabis testified before the state, including Stacey Linn and Jack Splitt, and Jennie Stormes on behalf of Jackson. The campaign worked. "Jack's Law" passed the state senate by a 35–0 vote and the house by a 56–9 vote. Governor Hickenlooper signed the bill into law in June of 2016.[8]

Unfortunately, Jack Splitt would not live long enough to really see the effects of his and his mother's activism. The 15-year-old, who friends and family described as a "charmer" and a "fighter," passed away in August of that year, leaving behind his mom, Stacey, and younger brother, Cooper. But Jack's legacy lives on, not only for pediatric patients in Colorado, who can now access their medicine legally at school, but also as an inspiration to students and their parents across the country.

In the years since Jack's Law passed in Colorado multiple parents across the U.S. have approached legislators or gone to court to fight for their children's right to receive legal medical cannabis at school. In the spring of 2018, Illinois parents Jim and Maureen Surin sued their daughter Ashley's school district to allow the 11-year-old to wear her CBD patch while at school. In April a federal judge issued an emergency order to allow the girl to return to school with her medicine.[9] While that order applied only to Ashley Surin, in August of that year Illinois Governor Bruce Rauner signed a law requiring schools to allow parents to administer prescribed cannabis to eligible children on campus.[10] Around the time Rauner signed the bill in Illinois a California family was also fighting for their child's right to medical cannabis at school. The Adams family took their school district to court to allow their kindergarten-age daughter to attend school with her medicine. In August a state court ruled in favor of the family, and the state legislature has recently passed a bill to allow school districts to create policies for medical marijuana on campus (the bill awaits the governor's signature).[11] If California's law passes, the state will join New Jersey (whose policy predates Colorado's), Colorado, Washington, Maine, and Illinois in allowing children to receive their marijuana medicine on campus. New Mexico and Florida are also considering policies. However, these laws and policies are a hodgepodge, with some states allowing school district policies but not requiring them and some allowing school nurses to administer the medication (a recent policy change in Colorado), while others require parents to come to school to administer the drug. Additionally, in many states the onus is left on the parents of special needs children to take these cases to court or to the legislature, a constant reinvention of the wheel that falls on the backs of these already-overburdened families. Medical marijuana in schools is just another of example of an area in which federal marijuana prohibition harms patients and their families alike.

Like Jennie Stormes and Stacey Linn, many of the activists in the fight for marijuana patients' rights in Colorado are parents, particularly moms. In fact, several groups, like CannaMoms, have formed just to support the mothers of cannabis patients and to advocate for their kids. These activist groups build upon years of marijuana activism in Colorado that set the stage not only for medical and recreational legalization but also made the state attractive for the first wave of medical marijuana refugees. Medical cannabis first became legal in Colorado in the year 2000 with the passing of Amendment 20. However, the Amendment did not set out policy, and the Department of Health (in closed door meetings with the DEA) decided to limit each medical marijuana caregiver (the person responsible for providing the cannabis) to five patients, severely handicapping the industry and its potential medical benefits.

Meanwhile, Brian Vicente was learning about marijuana policy from Professor K.K. DuVivier as a law student at the University of Denver on a Public Interest Scholarship. He had always known that he wanted to practice law to fight injustices, and as he learned about the racist and unjust practices involved in the War on Drugs he found his calling. When he graduated in 2004 he took a fellowship with the Marijuana Policy Project and soon founded Sensible Colorado, a nonprofit that would become one of the chief entities working on behalf of medical marijuana patients in Colorado. Sensible Colorado's campaigns included many direct actions such as protests, petitions to the health department, and even publicity stunts. But it was strategic litigation, led by Vicente, that would really set Colorado up as the benchmark for marijuana legalization.

In 2006 Vicente met Damien LaGoy, a medical marijuana patient suffering from AIDS and hepatitis C. Originally Vicente represented LaGoy when he was fined $500 by Denver police for possession of marijuana. When LaGoy told the officer that he was using marijuana to help with the symptoms of HIV, the officer retorted, "Is that any excuse to smoke pot?"[12] Denver eventually dropped the ticket when it became a publicity nightmare for the city. However, the following year Vicente agreed to continue to work with LaGoy on what would become a test case for Colorado's medical marijuana regulations. LaGoy wanted to see a caregiver named Dan Pope, but Pope already had five patients, the legal limit. Nevertheless, LaGoy applied to have Pope as his caregiver, and his application was rejected. He appealed, and it was rejected again.

Vicente and LaGoy sued the state of Colorado over what they stated was an arbitrary policy that infringed on patients' rights to receive their medicine legally. In a powerful day of testimony, LaGoy lined up his 50 prescription medications on the witness stand and stated, "I can't take any of these without medical marijuana." Without cannabis he was simply too nauseated to keep the pharmaceuticals down. Due to LaGoy's moving testimony and the fact that the caregiver limits were not written in the amendment but rather as an after-the-fact policy set up by the health department in secret meetings with the DEA, the policy was overturned. Caregivers could now have an unlimited number of patients, opening the door for retail marijuana establishments (more commonly known as dispensaries). Within two years there were more than 50 dispensaries in Colorado, and the health department decided again to try to limit the commercial distribution of medical marijuana by bringing back the five-patient limit for caregivers. This time, though, they had public hearings in order to get the Board of Health to sign off on the regulations. Vicente and Sensible Colorado once again opposed the regulation, and over 300 people showed up at the public hearing at Metro State University in Denver for eight hours of testimony. The board of health rejected the regulation, and, as Sensible Colorado stated, "the 'green rush' was born."[13]

As the number of dispensaries and registered patients in Colorado continued to grow, the state of Colorado and activist groups such as Sensible Colorado recognized the necessity for a state-regulated medical marijuana system. In 2010 the Colorado legislature enacted the Colorado

Medical Marijuana Code, "the most comprehensive system of medical marijuana distribution and regulation in the world," with the passage of SB 10–109 and HB 10–1284. Colorado thus became the first state to regulate marijuana commerce, setting up the Medical Marijuana Enforcement Division (which would later come to be known as the Marijuana Enforcement Division) and placing Colorado at the forefront of legal marijuana policy and commerce.[14]

Brian Vicente, Sensible Colorado, and other medical marijuana proponents set the ground for recreational legalization, which would come with the passing of Amendment 64 in 2012 with 55 percent of the vote. As Mason Tvert, communications director for the Marijuana Policy Project (MPP) states, "We would not be where we are in this state medicinally if it were not for Amendment 64." He claims that recreational legalization led to lesser stigma for marijuana users, an increase in patients' rights, especially for children and students, increased access to a variety of cannabis products, and progress in both technology and product quality. The story of full legalization that has led to these advancements starts back in 2004 with the deaths of two young Colorado college students.

In August of 2004 Samantha Spady drove from her hometown of Beatrice, Nebraska, to Fort Collins, Colorado, to start her sophomore year at Colorado State University. In high school Samantha, known as "Sam" to her friends and family, had been an honor roll student who was also the cheerleading captain, senior class president, and homecoming queen. She was also well liked at college, where she was majoring in business and was a "little sister" at Sigma Pi fraternity. On the fourth of September, a beautiful fall Saturday, Sam geared up for a night of partying with her friends. They first headed to a house party to watch the CU/CSU football game on TV. She started off with a couple of beers and a few shots of tequila before moving to the next party, where she consumed at least four or five more beers and some shots of vodka. At about 2:00 A.M. she and her friends found themselves at the Sigma Pi fraternity house, a familiar locale for Sam. She continued drinking for the next two hours, switching to straight vanilla-flavored vodka. By 4:30 A.M. she was so intoxicated that she could not stand up and did not respond when friends talked to her.[15] They helped her to a couch in a spare room of the house and left her there to "sleep it off." Samantha's body was not found until 6:20 that night when a fraternity member who lived off site was giving his mother a tour of the house. A blood test at the hospital after her death revealed a .436 percent blood-alcohol level, although the coroner said "it probably was higher when she was left there; her body would have continued to metabolize alcohol while she was unconscious."[16] A blood alcohol level above .35 is considered life threatening; drinkers will enter a coma and some will die at the .4 level, and .45 is the fatal blood-alcohol level for any human.[17]

Less than two weeks later and about 45 miles south, it was hazing night for the new pledges of Chi Psi fraternity at the University of Colorado, Boulder. On the evening of September 16 Gordon "Gordie" Bailey and 26 other prospective fraternity brothers, dressed in suits and ties for "bid night," were driven blindfolded into the Arapaho National Forest near Gold Hill, Colorado. They were told to drink "four handles of whiskey and six bottles of wine around a bonfire in 30 minutes." When they returned to the fraternity house Gordie was visibly intoxicated, and he passed out at around 11:00 P.M. He was placed on a couch, and "his brothers proceeded to write on his body with permanent markers—a fraternity ritual meant to embarrass brothers who pass out." Then, like Sam Spady, he was left to sleep it off. Nobody checked on him for almost ten hours, and his dead body was found face down on the floor the next morning.[18]

Samantha Spady and Gordie Bailey are just two of the many young people who die every year from binge drinking. So what do their deaths have to do with marijuana policy in Colorado? Well, in 2004 Mason Tvert and Steve Fox were developing a new campaign for the Marijuana Policy Project (MPP). Tvert had just finished working on campaigns in Arizona, highlighting candidates' positions on medical marijuana. Fox, who was the director of government relations for MPP, had worked with Tvert on the same campaigns. The two men had an idea for a new campaign called SAFER (Safer Alternatives for Enjoyable Recreation), which would attempt to change public attitudes by highlighting the relative safety of cannabis compared to alcohol. Cannabis scientists believe that it is impossible to die from consuming too much marijuana because the drug does not affect brain stem functions such as breathing. In fact, a user would have to consume 1,500 pounds in 15 minutes to get a lethal dose, clearly an impossibility.[19] Even the notoriously anti-cannabis

National Institute on Drug Abuse admits that no one has ever died from a marijuana overdose in the United States.[20] Compare that to the approximately six people who die every day in the U.S. from alcohol poisoning[21] or the over 49,000 Americans who died in 2017 from opioid overdose.[22] Studies at the time showed that approximately one-third of people thought that marijuana was safer than alcohol, approximately one-third thought that they were about equal in safety, and the rest thought that marijuana was more harmful than alcohol. Of the third who believed that marijuana was safer, 80 percent thought it should be legal. Of the other two-thirds 75 percent believed that it should remain illegal.[23] So Fox and Tvert believed that if they could convince people of the relative safety of cannabis they could pave the way toward political change.

Tvert and Fox had recently received funding from an MPP grant for the new campaign and were considering two possible states: Wisconsin and Colorado. These states were chosen because they had large university campuses, a large youth population, and a relative lack of initiatives around marijuana. Eventually, two events turned the tide in favor of Colorado: the deaths of Spady and Bailey. Because these two high-profile deaths occurred on the two major college campuses in Colorado, the time seemed right to begin a campaign based partly on alcohol's dangers. At first, the goal was simply to garner media coverage in an attempt to make people understand that marijuana was not the dangerous drug they had been taught it was. SAFER chapters were opened on the CU Boulder and CSU campuses to educate students. SAFER then did a poll on campus that showed that the majority of students believed that marijuana usage penalties were far too harsh in comparison with drinking penalties.

More and more students and Colorado residents began to come to the same realization that Mason Tvert had during his freshman year of college at the University of Richmond—a realization that would lead him into the world of marijuana activism—that marijuana is a less harmful drug than alcohol and should be regulated as such. Like Sam Spady and Gordy Bailey, Tvert had also suffered alcohol poisoning as a teenager. Fortunately, though, he survived, only having to spend a night in the hospital and receiving no legal consequences. But the following year at college he had a run in with law enforcement due to "alleged marijuana related activities." Just for smoking marijuana he was "harassed by law enforcement" and subpoenaed by a grand jury because of a drug task force fishing for information. He recalls that the experience "made me realize how ridiculous the laws were." And so, directly out of college, Tvert began working for the Marijuana Policy Project.

In Colorado in 2005 Fox and Tvert were experiencing success at the universities, so they decided to run the first decriminalization initiative in the city of Denver—a proposal to make personal possession of up to one ounce of cannabis legal for anyone over the age of 20. Although the men did not expect the initiative to pass, they thought it would garner a lot of free publicity for SAFER's cause. However, to their surprise, voters approved the measure, making Denver the first city in the nation to decriminalize marijuana possession. This victory led to various other initiatives, including a bill for statewide legalization the following year, which failed, with 40 percent of the vote in favor. Still, attitudes were changing, and SAFER passed another resolution in Denver in 2007 "making marijuana possession the city's lowest police priority."[24]

While the medical marijuana industry expanded greatly from 2007 to 2010, thanks largely to new regulations, Tvert was thinking of ways to continue the push for recreational legalization. He started a new campaign in conjunction with lawyer Brian Vicente called the Campaign to Regulate Marijuana Like Alcohol, drawing on SAFER's previous work comparing cannabis with the more dangerous, and legal, alcohol. In 2011 Vicente drafted Amendment 64, and the proposal made it onto the ballot. The amendment legalized possession of one ounce or less of marijuana for adults 21 years or older in the state of Colorado. It also regulated commercial sales through dispensaries and allowed the state to collect a voter-approved 15 percent excise tax on marijuana sales, with the first $40 million earmarked for public school construction in Colorado. Additionally, although it did not legalize personal sales it did allow cultivation of up to six plants at a time for adults over the age of 21.[25]

As we now know, the amendment passed in 2012 with 52.7 percent of the vote, making Colorado the first state to legalize recreational marijuana, followed closely by Washington state. And while medical marijuana was already a fast-growing industry at the time, it was really the passing and enactment of Amendment 64 that created the legal and social atmosphere for Colorado to be at the forefront of cannabis research and policy. Without the activism of early medical and recreational proponents like Mason Tvert and Brian Vicente, Colorado's cannabis policies and industry would not be what they are today—a magnet for patients from around the country and even the world. Still, it is the hard work of these patients and their families (like Stacey Linn and Jennie Stormes) who continue to push to improve Colorado's laws and policies for medical users.

Among these patients and activists is Teri Robnett, arguably one of the foremost leaders in patient activism in Colorado today. Teri is a Colorado native who graduated from the University of Colorado, Boulder, with a B.A. in psychology. She began her career working in the field of alternative medicine and was an activist for women's rights and civil rights. However, one day in 1987 would change the course of her life. Teri was driving home from her job in Boulder to the nearby town of Lafayette. As she was sitting at a stoplight in her small Mazda 323, she looked in her rearview mirror and saw a large car that did not appear to be slowing down. She remembers that she did what people are always told not to do: "I made a mistake and braced for the accident." She had her feet on the clutch and brake and her hands on the steering wheel, waiting for the impact. Her car was hit so hard that it slammed into the car in front of her.

Although Teri did not lose consciousness or break any bones, she had a massive amount of soft tissue damage. She had crunched every joint, so she developed problems in her neck, back, hips, knees, and ankles; all of her connective tissue was affected. For the first three weeks, she thought every day it couldn't "be more painful, and every day it was." After visiting a plethora of practitioners, she discovered that she had developed "fibrocytis," a condition now called fibromyalgia. Fibromyalgia is a medical disorder that involves widespread musculoskeletal pain accompanied by fatigue, sleep, and memory and mood issues. Some researchers think fibromyalgia amplifies painful sensations by affecting the way the brain processes pain signals.[26] The condition affects women more than men, and is often triggered, as with Teri's car accident, by a single traumatic event. Currently there is no cure for fibromyalgia, and patients can only attempt to control symptoms with pain killers, antidepressants, and other prescription drugs. Some patients do find a degree of relief from alternative therapies such as acupuncture and massage.

Over the next 20 years Teri tried everything for her disorder, but as with most fibromyalgia patients nothing worked very well. She remembers "the traditional medical side never gave [her] much relief." The "traditional medical side" basically consisted of prescription drugs for pain and inflammation—opiates and NSAIDs (nonsteroidal anti-inflammatory drugs), neither of which she ever really liked. In fact, she had a slight allergy to opiates, as they caused her to develop itching. She now considers this a lucky circumstance. Because she could not take them regularly, she did not develop the opiate addictions common among many chronic pain sufferers. She found the most relief from alternative practices including Pilates, acupuncture, nutrition, and craniosacral and chiropractic therapies; but even with these treatments, she lived constantly with pain, fatigue, insomnia, anxiety, and depression.

This all changed in 2009 when Teri took a job at a medical marijuana dispensary. Today she describes the experience as "eye opening," saying that her education about cannabis there was like being in a "language immersion program in a foreign country." Although she had used marijuana occasionally before, as soon as she learned of its medical benefits she decided to get on the registry and try it at medical doses. In contrast to pharmaceutical drugs, which she says have "been more harmful to me than any of the other stuff I have done," Teri credits using cannabis to treat her fibromyalgia with changing her life. Suddenly she had one drug that could treat not only her pain but also the insomnia, anxiety, and other symptoms that came with it. Additionally, she could control symptoms by changing strains and doses and not have to worry about the side effects of drug interactions. Her quality of life improved dramatically.

In 2012 Teri left her job at the dispensary to take care of her mother. However, like many other marijuana patients and families of patients, she found herself drawn into the politics surrounding cannabis. That year there was a bill in the state legislature that was attempting to combat driving under the influence of marijuana by establishing a hard limit of five nanograms of THC in the blood for a DUI. Teri knew from her own medicating that she would always be over that limit. In fact, because most patients need to use high doses of medical marijuana and they develop a tolerance for the drug, a high number of them would be over that limit even though they would not actually be impaired. Several other patients and activists recruited Teri to come to testify against the bill. Despite her activist background, it was her first time actually testifying before Congress, and she found the experience scary but exciting. She loved the idea that just by speaking out she could make a difference, and, in fact, she and the other activists were able to kill the bill twice that session.

Suddenly Teri became aware that there weren't many people speaking on behalf of medical marijuana patients and even fewer listening to what they had to say. There was still a misconception that patients were just wanting "to get high" and that marijuana was not truly a medicine for them. She decided that someone needed to change that perception and put a face to medical marijuana patients. That year, she founded the Cannabis Patients Alliance (CPA), a nonprofit alliance "of patients, families, organizations, businesses, advocates, activists and other supporters who work together to protect and advance the rights of patients who choose to use medical cannabis (marijuana) to treat whatever their condition may be." According to their website, CPA believes in "safe, legal, affordable access to medical marijuana in whatever way works best for the patient: home growing, caregivers, medical marijuana industry, retail marijuana industry or pharma, and access should be available through any and all of those means."

Like many patients who found themselves thrown into the world of cannabis activism, Teri Robnett and her organization have continued to work tirelessly for the rights of medical marijuana patients both in Colorado and throughout the country. In fact, today Teri is also known as Rx MaryJane and is considered one of the foremost experts on medical marijuana policy in Colorado. Since the passage of Amendment 64 much of Teri's work has focused on the unforeseen challenges to medical marijuana patients brought on by recreational legalization. Despite the many benefits for all users due to full legalization, the fact that Amendment 64 often directly contradicts Amendment 20, which legalized medical use, has led to some legal problems.

One of the issues Teri has been working to address is the fact that there is a constant push to combine medical and recreational use and policy. As Teri notes, "patients' needs are just not the same as the needs of recreational users." One aspect of this issue was a bill in 2017 to limit plant counts for home grows. HB 1220 reduced the quantity of plants that could be grown by patients unless there was already a county or city regulation in place. Recreational users are limited to growing six plants per person or 12 per household, while medical users previously could grow up to 99 plants with a doctor's recommendation. Lawmakers introduced HB 1220 in attempts to limit illegal grows and the funneling of marijuana out of state and into the black market. Under this premise the bill was originally proposed with a limit of 12 plants per patient. However, Teri Robnett, along with other patients' rights advocates,

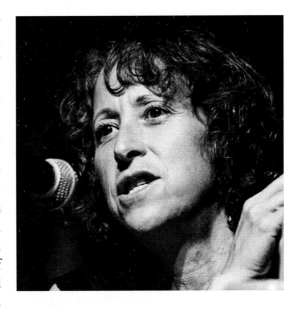

After finding that cannabis effectively controlled her fibromyalgia, Teri Robnett became a statewide advocate for medical marijuana patients in Colorado. Here she testifies in 2014 on a state panel (courtesy Greg Duran).

argued for higher limits for medical users. She stated that oftentimes patients require many more than 12 plants in order to make the amount of medicine they need. While they would still be able to buy medicinal marijuana at a dispensary, this is far more expensive than growing one's own and many patients live a long way from any dispensary. Essentially, proponents of the bill argued that the new regulations would "re-criminalize" medical users. Due to their lobbying, the bill was amended to up the limit to 16 plants. Later, the Senate Judiciary Committee amended the bill again, upping the limit to 24 plants if the patient/grower registered the grow with the state. While this is not an ideal situation for patients, advocates were pleased that they were able to double the originally proposed limits and also were able to get wording in the bill to exclude seedlings from plant counts. Additionally, the bill specifies that local ordinances on plant counts overrule the state limits, whether they are lower or higher.[27]

In addition to problems with regulations and laws at the state level, many issues surrounding legalization arise from the discrepancy between Colorado's laws and the federal law. For many years medical marijuana businesses worked in a gray area, protected by individual state laws yet open to raids by the Drug Enforcement Administration (DEA). After years of raids under the Bush administration (particularly in the state of California), President Obama asserted the following during his 2008 campaign; "I'm not going to be using Justice Department resources to try to circumvent state laws on this issue."[28] In February 2009, after Obama's election, Attorney General Eric Holden announced that the DEA would end its raids on state-approved medical marijuana businesses. Six months later the U.S. Department of Justice (DOJ) formalized this position in a memo that became known as the "Ogden Memo" after Deputy Attorney General David Ogden. In the memo the DOJ announced that prosecutorial priorities would not target "individuals whose actions are in clear and unambiguous compliance with existing state laws providing for the medical use of marijuana."[29]

While the Ogden Memo provided reassurance for medical marijuana patients and businesses, it was only three years before the Justice Department began to crack down on medical marijuana suppliers in legal states like California, Washington, and Montana. In fact, raids and arrests for medical marijuana rose to a level far exceeding those under Obama's predecessor, George W. Bush. The crackdowns were apparently spurred on by a perception in the DOJ that medical marijuana had gotten "out of hand" and that the industry had been "hijacked by profiteers."[30] Perhaps because Colorado's medical cannabis industry had more defined regulations at the state level (rather than local-level regulations like those in California), the state was spared the worst of the raids. The new hard-line approach was formalized in a memo to U.S. district attorneys in June of 2011 by David Ogden's successor, James Cole. The Cole memo laid out priorities for federal enforcement of marijuana laws and completely contradicted Holden's statements from 2009. The memo promised no protection for individuals or businesses operating under state law, declaring that the feds could go after "[p]ersons who are in the business of cultivating, selling or distributing marijuana, and those who knowingly facilitate such activities ... regardless of state law."[31]

This turnaround in federal policy not only set up a clash between state and federal regulations but also paved the way for a new round of raids. Because there no longer seemed to be a distinction between good and bad operators, the feds indiscriminately began to raid medical dispensaries, driving patients into the black market or making it impossible for them to get the medicine they needed. One dispensary that was closed down was Humboldt Medical Supply in Humboldt County, a state-permitted dispensary that gave free marijuana to elderly patients and "was seen as a model of compliance with local regulations."[32] Northstone Organics Collective, a licensed Mendocino medical marijuana cooperative owned by Matthew Cohen, despite being praised by the Mendocino County sheriff for "scrupulous adherence to the rules," was raided by the DEA in October. Federal agents with assault rifles destroyed all of Mr. Cohen's property, including plants that were meant to provide medicine for the co-op's 1,700 members.[33] These raids were part of a new crackdown on medical marijuana in the U.S. even as more states legalized, and polls at the time showed that over 70 percent of Americans favored medical marijuana legalization.[34] In 2012 *Rolling Stone's* Tim Dickinson noted, "The Obama administration has quietly unleashed a multi-agency crackdown on medical cannabis that goes far beyond anything undertaken by George W. Bush. The feds are busting growers who operate in full compliance with state laws, vowing to seize the property of anyone who dares to even rent to legal pot dispensaries, and threatening to imprison state employees responsible for regulating medical marijuana." By 2013 Americans for Safe Access reported that the DEA had carried out 270 medical marijuana raids under Obama, threatening access to medicine for 750,000 cannabis patients in California alone.[35]

At this point, fed up with the DOJ and DEA's heavy-handed tactics, state governments began to resist. The Rohrabacher-Farr Amendment (initially known as the Hinchey-Rohrabacher Amendment) was legislation first introduced to Congress in 2003 by U.S. representatives Maurice Hinchey, Dana Rohrabacher, and Sam Farr. The amendment prohibits the Justice Department from spending funds to interfere with the implementation of state medical marijuana laws.[36] The bill failed six times over the next decade but by 2014, propelled by increasing resentment over federal intervention in state marijuana laws, it passed as part of an omnibus spending bill, providing historic protection for legal cannabis patients. However, the bill must be renewed each year, so this protection is fragile.

Around this same time, states with medical marijuana (and some, like Colorado, with legal recreational marijuana) were facing another hurdle due to federal regulations—banking. *Rolling Stone* reported on it at the time: "The federal war on medical marijuana has locked pot dispensaries out of the banking system—especially in Colorado, home to the nation's second-largest market for medicinal cannabis. Top banks—including Chase, Wells Fargo and Bank of America—are refusing to do business with state-licensed dispensaries, for fear of federal prosecution for money-laundering and other federal drug crimes." Thus, Representatives Jared Polis and Ed Perlmutter from Colorado cosponsored HB2652, introduced in 2013. The bill, entitled Marijuana Businesses Access to Banking Act, aimed "to create protections for depository institutions that provide financial services to marijuana-related businesses."[37] However, it died in Congress. The bill was reintroduced in 2015 but again was not enacted.

Meanwhile, although it is not illegal for banks to have marijuana businesses as clients, many still are not willing to take the risk. In 2014 the U.S. Department of Justice and the Treasury Department's Financial Crimes Enforcement Network (FinCEN) released a joint statement with guidelines for banks wishing to provide services to legal cannabis businesses. The seven-page memo outlined ways in which banks could help the federal government uncover illegal activity while assuring they are banking with marijuana businesses that abide by local laws. While the memo gave the green light for marijuana banking, it also required banks to submit a Suspicious Activity Report (SAR) on any marijuana businesses they serviced and also provided a list of more than 20 "red flags" that could show federal law violations.[38] Although the cannabis industry welcomed the report (running cash-based businesses is undesirable for a variety of reasons), many banks were still unwilling to get involved in the gray area between federal and state law. As the American Bankers Association said, the "guidance" "does not change the fact that possession and distribution of marijuana is still illegal under federal law. And, the Department of Justice emphasizes that financial transactions connected with marijuana businesses can still form the basis for prosecution, putting any bank on notice that the risks are high."[39] Because the

FinCEN memo is guidance rather than law, Representative Perlmutter continues to fight for legal banking for marijuana businesses. In 2017, with representatives from Washington and Alaska, he introduced a new version of his previous bill, renamed Secure and Fair Enforcement Banking Act (SAFE Banking Act), or HR 2215. Until such federal legislation is enacted, marijuana businesses and their customers will continue to face risks. As Perlmutter states, "First and foremost, this is an issue of public safety. Not only are the proprietors at risk, but the employees and customers are also at risk of serious and violent crimes. It is estimated that 40 percent of the marijuana-related businesses in Colorado are unbanked. This means hundreds of millions of dollars in cash are moving around the streets of Colorado."[40]

Until federal law catches up with state laws, medical marijuana users will continue to face struggles in obtaining their medicine, and the industry will continue in its struggles to provide for them. After over one hundred years of prohibition, medical marijuana laws are still in the process of being worked out. As Mason Tvert from the Marijuana Policy Project notes, alcohol prohibition ended almost 100 years ago and we are still fine-tuning alcohol laws in this country. As we continue to modify laws around medical marijuana, it will be imperative for patients to step forward and work with activists and lawmakers to ensure that the changes made benefit them rather than limiting their access to the medicine they need.

CHAPTER 3

Providing Hope

Vicki Pletka was 26 weeks pregnant with her daughter Lilith (Lily) when the doctors told her and her wife, Rosie Wirth, that their baby had several rare brain malformations. Vicki was advised to terminate the pregnancy, and doctors said that if Lily did survive the birth she would have no quality of life—would not walk or talk and likely would not make it to her first birthday. Vicki and Rosie decided to go ahead with the pregnancy, and today Lily is a happy and thriving five-year-old, thanks in large part to Haleigh's Hope CBD oil, produced by Jason Cranford in Boulder County, Colorado. The road to where Lily and her mothers are today has not been an easy one, however. Like many other refugees, the Pletka-Wirths faced a long and costly battle before receiving the medicine Lily needed. But their story is more than indicative of the important role played by growers and producers in Colorado's medical marijuana boom.

Lily Pletka-Wirth was born in early 2011 in Wisconsin. She was immediately diagnosed with four brain malformations: agenesis of the corpus callosum (a complete or partial absence of the corpus callosum), ventriculomegaly (when the fluid-filled structures called lateral ventricles in the brain are too large), colpocephaly (disproportionate enlargement of the occipital horns of the lateral ventricles in the brain), and hydrocephalus (fluid on the brain).[1] She also had two genetic mutations (SCN2A & GRIN2B). Doctors said that she was the only child in the world with this combination of brain disorders, and to this day Vicki calls her "my unicorn." Lily immediately began having seizures after she was born, and she was soon having around 100 a day. Still, it was three years before doctors diagnosed her with Dravet's syndrome. Like the parents of other children who eventually end up trying cannabis, Vicki and Rosie spent the first four years of Lily's life in and out of the hospital, desperately trying to find treatments to allow her to thrive. Yet she continued to have dozens of daily seizures and also suffered from autism, bradycardia (abnormally slow heart), developmental delays, failure to thrive, asthma, allergies, celiac disorder, and various other issues.

Because of her daughter's rare condition, Vicki was always doing research, always looking for something that would help to alleviate her symptoms. In 2014 she heard the story of then-four-year-old Haleigh Cox. From Georgia, Haleigh is now seven. She suffers from Lennox-Gastaut Syndrome and Cerebral Palsy. Like Lily, by the time she was three years old she was having over 100 seizures every day. Her parents heard about the success of Charlotte's Web for epileptic children, so in 2014 her mom moved to Colorado with her to seek treatment. Because there was a shortage of the high–CBD Charlotte's Web, available through the Realm of Caring, and a long wait list for the oil, she contacted Jason Cranford, another medical marijuana provider. He too had a high–CBD oil, which he provided to the family. Within weeks, the little girl's

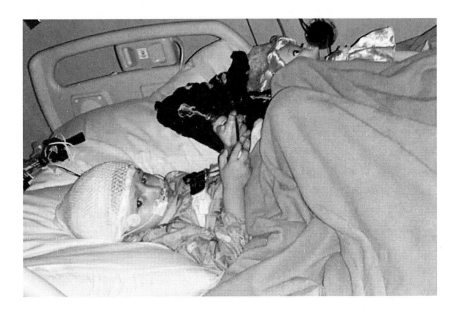

Before starting to use cannabis oil Lily Pletka-Wirth was having more than 100 seizures a day, despite a variety of pharmaceuticals and other treatments (courtesy Vicki Pletka).

seizures were drastically reduced.[2] When Vicki heard the story, she too decided to try Cranford's oil, which by now he had named "Haleigh's Hope."

Technically Vicki should have been able to have Haleigh's Hope shipped to her home in Wisconsin. However, at that time, Cranford wasn't yet shipping his product. Additionally, although CBD-only oil is legal in the state under "Lydia's Law," the reality is that, like many states where medical marijuana or CBD oil is legal, the law is essentially useless. At the time, it was legal to possess CBD-only products in the state, but it was illegal to produce them or transport them into the state and few, if any, doctors were willing to prescribe cannabis. So Lily's doctor recommended that the family move to Colorado.

Despite everything they had been through, it was not easy for the Pletka-Wirths to make the decision to move the family to Colorado. Vicki had always been the "square" in her group of friends. She doesn't drink or do drugs, and even after doing the research on cannabis she was skeptical. Her extended family also did not believe it would work; they snidely called it a "miracle medicine." Additionally, moving would break the family up, as Vicki had two children living with their father. Indeed, she ended up losing visitation rights with them because of her daughter's use of medical marijuana. Still, Vicki had always been open to alternative medicine and was desperate to do whatever it took to help her daughter's rare condition. She recalls, "I was a mom who held my child seizing hundreds of times a day and begged and pleaded with her to start breathing again, to please stop seizing. I begged, 'Don't leave me. Please come back to me.' At that point I was willing to try anything."

Thus, in the beginning of April 2015, Vicki and Rosalinda had a 30-day yard sale to sell almost everything they owned. They decided that as soon as they raised $5,000 they would leave for Colorado. Around that time, the local media picked up the story and they were soon receiving dozens of donations on a GoFundMe page. Before long they had raised over $10,000, and they were able to move on May 9, 2015. Like many other medical marijuana families, they moved to Colorado Springs and started Lily on Haleigh's Hope oil as soon as possible. Change happened quickly. In the first three days she continued to seize, but they were seeing decreases in her seizure activity. Vicki kept explaining away the changes as "coincidence." However, on day three Lily started "spouting out sentences on her own and random words." Before this, she had been considered nonverbal. She would imitate words, but even though she was four years old she could not formulate her own thoughts. Vicki remembers thinking, *Why is my kid talking? My kid doesn't talk!*

Within her first week on the oil Lily had her first day without a seizure. Vicki and Rosalinda kept "waiting for the other shoe to drop," not really believing it could be working so well. But, even though they were also weaning her off of her pharmaceuticals at the time, she continued to improve. Her cognitive functioning rapidly progressed, and she soon hit two weeks without a seizure. Her moms had to admit that the cannabis oil was working. These days, Lily still has occasional seizures, but her condition is hugely improved since before cannabis. The longest she has gone without a seizure is 26 days, and when she does have seizures they are quick drop seizures that are not nearly as severe as before. THC rescue meds rubbed directly on her gums will take her right out of a tonic clonic seizure, and with her once-daily dose

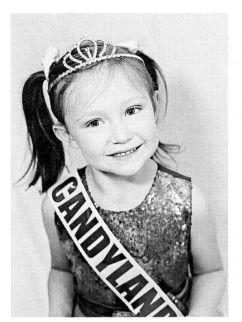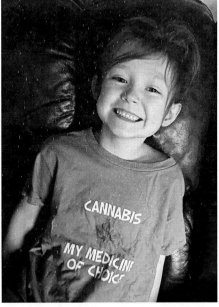

After starting high–CBD cannabis oil Lily Pletka-Wirth's seizures dropped by 95 percent. Today she is a thriving and happy little girl (courtesy Vicki Pletka).

of CBD oil her overall seizure rate has reduced by 95 percent. Cognitively, she went from an 18-month-old level to a 3½-year-old level in one year. Also, before starting Haleigh's Hope, Lily had extremely low growth hormone levels; she was not really gaining weight even with formula and a tube. However, after starting the oil she began gaining weight and her growth hormone levels evened out at normal. As Vicki says, the whole situation is a "Cinderella story!"

About a year after Lily began taking cannabis oil the family took a secret trip back to Wisconsin to visit their family. Because it is illegal to transport cannabis over state lines and because of the wide difference between state laws, it is very dangerous for medical marijuana patients to leave their state. In fact, many patients described feeling like "prisoners." The situation is even worse for parents of pediatric patients, since they could have their children taken away if they were found to have cannabis in their system. Some people never leave; others do so secretly. When the Pletka-Wirths got back to Wisconsin, the family members who had been skeptical that the drug could work had their minds changed when they saw the remarkable improvement in Lily. Even Rosalinda's mom, a retired police officer, had to admit that the cannabis was working. The doctors and nurses back in Wisconsin were also blown away by Lily's improvement. Nothing changes minds about the effectiveness of cannabis as medicine like seeing firsthand the positive benefits that it can have for patients. Meanwhile, the Pletka-Wirths, although they miss Wisconsin, have no regrets about moving to Colorado. While it is hard being away from their family and their other kids, the improvements in Lily are worth it. As Vicki points out, "She gets to tell us she loves us. When she's mad, she gets to tell us she's mad at us." As a mom, Vicki says, she "could want nothing more."

As Lily Pletka-Wirth's story makes clear, legalizing CBD oil (or even medical marijuana in general) is no guarantee for treatment within a particular state. Without policies around producing and distributing the medicine, many laws have no teeth at all. In fact, while there are currently 46 states with medical marijuana laws on the books (plus the District of Columbia, Guam, and Puerto Rico), very few have fully functioning systems. Of those 46 states, 13 only allow use of "low THC, high cannabidiol (CBD) products for medical reasons in limited situations or as a legal defense" (ncsl.org). Because they don't allow THC medicines, these states are not considered to have comprehensive medical marijuana programs. Of the remaining 33 states, eight, including Florida, Pennsylvania, and West Virginia, are considered "not yet functional," meaning that policies are not in place and the law is not yet operative. Others, like Alaska, do not allow for dispensaries as part of state law, making it very difficult for patients to get the medicines they need. Some states, like New Jersey, do not allow for home grows, making the medicine difficult to obtain and prohibitively expensive for many patients.[3]

Colorado's law, while not the first in the country, was the first to create a regulated dispensary system and is also at the forefront of patients' rights. As part of its pioneering legal position, Colorado is home to many growers and producers who are in the vanguard of innovating new cannabis strains and products. While the most famous of these is undoubtedly the Stanley brothers (creators of high–CBD strain Charlotte's Web) due to their appearance on Sanjay Gupta's CNN special *Weed*, there are many other growers and producers working to create new product and help the many patients who are moving to the state.

One of the most prominent of this group of innovative producers is Jason Cranford, owner and founder of Haleigh's Hope oil and the Flowering Hope foundation. Cranford, originally from Georgia, moved to California to work in the cannabis industry. In 2007 he was living in Humboldt County and cultivating for the medical industry. After reading Raphael Mechoulam's studies involving cannabinoids, he decided to try and cultivate a higher CBD strain of marijuana. He travelled around Northern California collecting plants to test them for a high CBD genetic. Eventually his search led him to Colorado, where he gathered around 100 plants and found the high–CBD genetic he was looking for. He hired a biochemist to test the plants and found that one particular plant had the highest CBD levels in the world at the time. That original strain was "Bubblegum Kush," and by in-breeding and selective breeding he was able to bring the CBD/THC ratio from 1–1 to 20–1 over time. This new strain became Haleigh's Hope.

In 2009, after learning of new licensing laws for growers, Cranford decided to relocate to Colorado. He jumped headfirst into the growing industry—building grow rooms, consulting on cultivation, and founding his own companies. Today he is the owner of South Park Pharma, an organic wholesale marijuana cultivation facility, and the codeveloper of

Cannatol RX, a cannabis rescue nasal spray. He is a grower and caregiver for approximately 250 patients and he works as a general contractor specializing in the construction of cannabis cultivation facilities. In addition, he is an outspoken advocate for patients' rights in Colorado and throughout the country and founded the nonprofit Flowering Hope Foundation to "facilitate safe access to life changing medication to those that suffer from multiple ailments."[4]

Around the same time he move to Colorado, Cranford also became more intimately involved with medical cannabis when, like many others, he witnessed the power of the plant firsthand. He was approached by the father of a four-year-old terminal brain cancer patient, asking him if he had any oil to help the child. He decided to donate 1:1 CBD: THC oil to the family. The little girl ended up living and beating cancer. Cranford recalls, "This changed me mentally and spiritually with my views on medicinal cannabis. It was never a hobby to me after this—it became a responsibility and a mission."[5] Cranford quietly began developing high–CBD oils and providing them to families in need.

Meanwhile, another high–CBD strain was being grown outside of Colorado Springs by six brothers—Joel, Jesse, Jon, Jordan, Jared, and Josh Stanley. Other small-scale growers were also developing similar strains at the time, but few of them were aware of the large potential market for the products. Charming and media-ready, the Stanley brothers were the first to respond when the news outlets arrived to cover this new phenomenon. After appearing on Sanjay Gupta's *Weed* special, along with other mainstream media outlets, the Stanley brothers, with their Charlotte's Web oil, became the faces of medical marijuana in Colorado. In addition, Paige Figi and Heather Jackson, mothers of two patients helped by the oil, along with Amanda Stanley, Joel Stanley's wife, formed a nonprofit called Realm of Caring (ROC) to connect potential patients with the medicine. Thus, dozens of families heard about the powers of Charlotte's Web through the CNN special, researched the Realm of Caring online, and soon made their way to Colorado to try the oil. Unfortunately, the Stanley brothers were not ready for this influx of new patients, and demand for their product soon outpaced supply. By 2014 there were 12,000 people around the country on the wait-list to receive Charlotte's Web, with "only 350 or so patients, mostly children, actually receiving oil made from the strain."

Jason Cranford, who was still running a relatively small operation, offered to step in and help some of the patients on the wait-list, and soon he became the second largest provider in Colorado of high–CBD cannabis oil to pediatric patients. Even as it grew, Cranford's business remained basically a grassroots operation, working on a different model than many other large cannabis oil providers. He operates as a basic caregiver, having a few employees who help him make his oil, which he then provides directly to patients. He does not sell his oil out of his recreational dispensaries because he believes it would be too difficult and expensive for his patients. Additionally, to address the issue of high costs for patients, he formed the nonprofit Flowering Hope Foundation in 2015. Unlike Realm of Caring, which primarily serves as patient support and conducts lobbying, Flowering Hope is a 501c3 that takes donations and has fundraisers and then uses that money to provide Haleigh's Hope for patients in need. Recipients need to prove that they are low income, and then the foundation steps in and covers the manufacturing costs. Flowering Hope also includes patient education as part of its mission and does seminars around the country at medical cannabis conferences and symposiums. Possibly most important, given the sometimes prohibitively high cost of cannabis medicines, Cranford provides clones of his plants to patients free of charge.

Allowing patients to grow their own medicine is an extremely important facet of patients' rights and is what differentiates grassroots providers like Cranford from large corporate providers and, significantly, the pharmaceutical industry. The pharmaceutical industry's involvement in and relationship with medical cannabis and marijuana laws is both complicated and controversial. Many patients and activists blame the industry and its influence on the FDA for the federal government's glacial speed in reassessing marijuana and its Schedule I status. Not surprisingly, patients who have gotten to the point of using cannabis for their illnesses (and particularly the parents of pediatric patients) have a deep distrust of the medical establishment and the pharmaceuticals they prescribe. In my interviews I heard dozens of stories of terrible reactions and side effects from prescription drugs, ranging from rage behaviors to organ trouble to breathing issues. Coltyn Turner, who suffered from Crohn's disease, was even told by doctors that he would eventually develop leukemia if he continued on the strong immunosup-

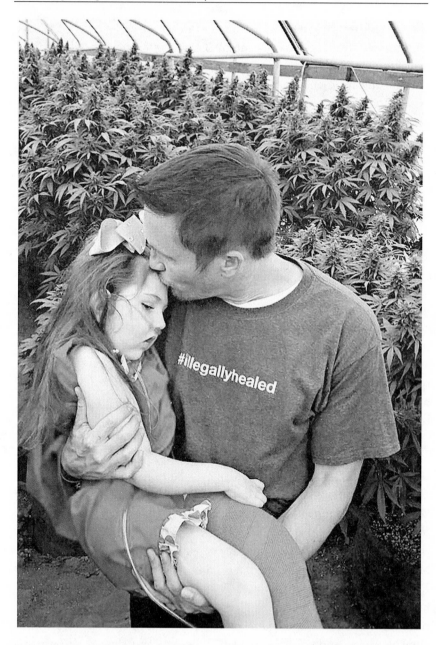

Jason Cranford holds Haleigh Cox in front of "Haleigh's Hope" plants—the high–CBD strain of cannabis he developed and named after the four-year-old Cox, whose seizures were controlled by the high–CBD oil. Cox is now a brand ambassador for Cranford's company.

pressant drugs he was taking for his disorder. Few, if any, doctors recommended cannabis for these patients while they were struggling with horrible effects from (and often addictions to) prescribed drugs, demonstrating the detrimental effects of a system that categorically favors pharmaceuticals.

Cannabis patients often learn the hard way that pharmaceuticals are not always the panacea that the medical establishment presents them as. This is not to say that doctors do not want what is best for their patients, but the amount of money involved in the pharmaceutical industry and inherent conflicts of interest between the FDA and pharmaceutical companies should give patients pause when considering their prescriptions. For example, while the pharmaceutical industry is responsible for the development of medicines to save lives and alleviate suffering, it is also an industry that generates higher profit margins than any other. U.S. pharmaceutical company Pfizer, the largest drug company in the world based on revenue, had a 42 percent profit margin in 2014. Compare this to the highest profit margins in other industries: 29 percent for banking, 24 percent for oil and gas, 18 percent for media and 10 percent for the automobile industry. These huge profit margins have led many to accuse the drug companies of profiteering at the expense of human health and lives. In fact, some drugs can cost more than $100,000 for a full course.[6]

Unethical price gouging made the news in 2015 when Martin Shkreli, hedge fund manager and CEO of Turing Pharmaceuticals, raised the cost of Daraprim 5,000 percent, from $13.50 a pill to $750 a pill. Daraprim is the only medicine available to treat toxoplasmosis, an infection caused by feline parasites that can cause birth defects in humans. It is also used in treatment for HIV, malaria, and some cancers.[7] In 2016 the drug company Mylan was hit with a class action racketeering lawsuit after it raised the price of its EpiPen 548 percent beginning in 2007. The EpiPen is commonly used to treat a potentially fatal allergic reaction known as anaphylaxis. About 3.4 million Americans a year are prescribed an EpiPen, including parents of children with severe nut, bee, and soy allergies who must carry the pen with them as a lifesaving measure in case of serious reactions. However, these patients must now pay $600 out of pocket for two EpiPens versus $100 for the two-pack in 2007.[8] Given the proliferation of price hikes on a variety of lifesaving medications it is no wonder that the public has grown wary of pharmaceutical companies.

Drug companies defend the high price of their medicines by pointing to the costs of research and development. In fact, a 2014 study by the Tufts Center for the Study of Drug Development (CSDD) found that it cost approximately $2.6 billion to develop a prescription drug that gains market approval.[9] Additionally, on average, only three out of ten drugs that are launched end up being profitable, and some don't even make it to market. Yet, a look at drug company statistics shows that these companies spend far more on marketing their drugs than they do on research and development (R&D). In fact, in 2013 U.S. company Johnson & Johnson spent $8.2 billion on R&D but over twice that, $17.5 billion, on sales and marketing. Despite the large outlay on research and development, the company made $71.3 billion in total revenue, with a profit of $13.8 billion (19 percent profit margin). Numbers are similar across the pharmaceutical industry, demonstrating that R&D costs are not responsible for high consumer prices.[10]

Drug companies also argue that they have to charge high prices because they have a limited time to make money off of drugs due to patent laws. It is true that patents are usually awarded for 20 years, but since up to 12 of those years can be used on research and development, companies are often left with less than ten years to sell their product before the formula is opened up to generic drug companies. Once that happens, sales can drop by over 90 percent. However, drug companies go to great lengths to extend their patents—a process that is known as "evergreening."[11] They do this by creating new formulations that either change a few ingredients in the original drug or combine two drugs to create a new product. So while it is certainly expensive to research and develop new drugs and companies have relatively short windows to sell those drugs before they lose their patents, they are still making huge profits.

What does all of this have to do with medical marijuana? It is important to explore the workings of the legal drug industry in the United States in order, first, to understand why marijuana continues to be illegal despite its obvious medical benefits, and, second, to understand how to create a nationwide medical marijuana industry that is profitable while still benefiting patients. As explained previously, there are a variety of reasons why marijuana was made illegal in the early 20th century, and the medical establishment quickly jumped on board with policy makers in banning the drug. Since then, federal research has been limited on cannabis due mostly to its Schedule I status but also because of the complex relationships between the DEA, the FDA, and pharmaceutical companies. Additionally, most doctors tend to know very little about the drug, since it is not taught in medical school and even in legal states many are afraid to recommend it due to its Schedule I status (since it is a federally restricted substance, MDs might risk losing their licenses if they prescribe it). Many doctors learn about recent medications from the pharmaceutical company representatives who visit their offices or host continuing education conferences with information on, and samples of, new drugs.

While the medical marijuana industry lacks reps who can promote the drug to doctors, the public has known for many years that the pharmaceutical industry markets directly to physicians. In fact, data on payments to doctors in the U.S. has recently become available due to the "Sunshine Act," a provision of the Affordable Care Act. Now the Centers for Medicare and Medicaid Services must publish all payments over $10 made from medical companies to doctors and hospitals. A recent study in *JAMA: The Journal of the American Medical Association (Internal Medicine)* used this data to find a controversial association between industry payments to doctors and prescribing rates. The researchers looked at the association between doctors' pharmaceutical industry-sponsored meals (accounting for 80 percent of the total amount of payments) and their rates of prescribing the promoted drug to Medicare beneficiaries. They found "receipt of industry-sponsored meals was associated with an increased rate of prescribing the brand-name medication that was being promoted. The findings represent an association, not a cause-and-effect relationship."[12]

When patients visit a doctor they expect to be recommended or prescribed the best treatment for their condition. Unfortunately, pharmaceutical industry practices would seem to impair physicians' objectivity in making decisions about drugs. In addition to paying for meals, conference trips, and the like, drug companies also give doctors free samples to hand out to patients. Combine this influence with the multimillion dollar, direct-to-consumer marketing of such drugs, and it is clear that drug companies have far too much influence over which drugs doctors choose to prescribe and which drugs Americans choose to take. It is no surprise then that in states where medical marijuana is legal the majority of physicians still do not recommend cannabis, even when it may be the best treatment for a patient's condition. Medical schools don't teach about marijuana, and companies producing cannabis medicine don't have field reps visiting physicians' offices to hand out samples, pay for elaborate meals, and leave pamphlets about the drug. Given these facts, it's no wonder that prescription drugs are still the treatment of choice for most physicians, even when their side effects may be crippling. Patients in legal medical marijuana states are dependent on producers and caregivers like Jason Cranford and a few doctors and researchers like Alan Shackelford to provide them with knowledge about and recommendations for cannabis. Those in Colorado's thriving cannabis industry, along with a corps of open-minded doctors, have thus been able to counter the heavy influence of the pharmaceutical industry and create a state where medical cannabis is a real option for patients, attracting prospective patients from around the country.

Of course, given the fact that the pharmaceutical industry is such an influential and integral part of the medical establishment, many patients and physicians alike would prefer to see cannabis medicinals become part of the industry. As a pharmaceutical, medical marijuana would be more thoroughly researched to document safety and efficacy and production would adhere to Current Good Manufacturing Practices (CGMP), resulting in products meeting established quality requirements such as consistency and strength. Additionally, the drug would possibly be covered by insurance companies, Medicare/Medicaid, and the VA, potentially alleviating the issue of prohibitive costs. In fact, synthetic forms of marijuana have been legally available in the U.S. for years. The first cannabis-based drug to be developed and approved was Marinol (generic name dronabinol), a synthetic Delta-9 THC manufactured by Unimed Pharmaceuticals. Marinol was developed as a treatment for nausea and vomiting for patients in cancer treatment, as an appetite stimulant for AIDS patients, and as a painkiller for multiple sclerosis patients. The United States FDA first approved it as a Schedule I drug for nausea in 1985 and then approved it as an appetite stimulant in 1992. It was reclassified as a Schedule III drug in 1999.[13]

Currently, the British drug company GW Pharmaceuticals has taken the lead in developing marijuana-based medications. Unlike Marinol, GW Pharma's products are actually plant-derived rather than being wholly synthetic. The company developed Sativex, the world's first prescription medicine derived from the marijuana plant, in 2010. The drug was originally approved and launched in the UK for neuropathic pain and spasticity associated with multiple sclerosis. It was also approved for pain treatment for patients with advanced stages of cancer. Since then it has been approved in 29 countries around the world, not including the United States. While the drug has undergone trials in the U.S. for many years, it has yet to pass out of clinical trial phases. GW Pharma's most recent product is Epidiolex, a liquid formulation of plant-derived CBD, the cannabinoid in Charlotte's Web and Haleigh's Hope that has been found effective in treating various early onset, treatment-resistant seizure disorders. Epidiolex was approved by the FDA in 2018 after preliminary trials showed promising signs of efficacy.[14]

While there are many benefits to having cannabis medications developed by pharmaceutical companies and licensed and approved by the FDA, many, if not most, patients and advocates do not want the industry to take over sole production of the drug. For almost all medical advocates in the U.S., and even worldwide, retaining the ability to grow one's own plants and to have access to full-plant medicine are key components of patients' rights. One reason for this is that synthetic and single cannabinoid medicines have not been found to be as effective as whole-plant therapy. While Marinol has been available by prescription since the 1980s, many cancer and AIDS patients still chose to illicitly search out whole-plant marijuana, which they find more effectively manages their symptoms. Although peer-reviewed studies have shown increased pain relief for patients using dronabinol versus a placebo, many patients who tried both the synthetic THC pill and smoked marijuana found that the pill was not nearly as effective in alleviating symptoms.[15] One 56-year-old patient who was prescribed Marinol for chronic nausea and vomiting due to gastroparesis reported, "I felt no relief.... I felt nothing. It might as well be M&Ms." Another patient quoted in the same study was prescribed Marinol for his multiple sclerosis. He described the difference between smoked marijuana and the synthetic pills: "If I smoke a joint, the tremors go away most times before the joint is gone. It makes my life a little easier." Marinol, by contrast, "didn't really do much of anything for me."[16] These anecdotal accounts are backed up by prescribing doctors all over the country and could partly explain why, 30 years after being legally approved, Marinol remains far less popular than whole-plant medical marijuana.

There are a variety of reasons why pharmaceutical marijuana is not usually found to be as effective as the whole-plant variety. For one, smoked or vaporized cannabis offers faster relief than oral ingestion of the drug. As Dr. Mitch Earleywine, an associate professor of clinical psychology at the State University of New York at Albany writes, "[One] problem with Marinol is that it's orally administered. Therefore, it takes longer to work than cannabis inhaled from a vaporizer. (Usually 90 minutes at best rather than 15 seconds—a meaningful amount of time to the nauseated.) In addition, folks who are vomiting can't hold down the pills."[17] Also, all of the marijuana-based drugs that are currently developed contain only one cannabinoid—THC or CBD. As mentioned previously, the marijuana plant is known to contain over 110 cannabinoids, with more being discovered all the time. It is currently unknown how the various compounds in marijuana work together, but it is known that they seem to have an "entourage effect," being more effective in combination than alone. One recent peer-reviewed medical study out of Israel confirmed the superior therapeutic value of whole-plant CBD extract versus synthetic, single molecule cannabidiol. The researchers from the Hebrew University of Jerusalem studied the two drugs in mice, and concluded "the therapeutic synergy observed with plant extracts results in the requirement for a lower amount of active components, with consequent reduced adverse effects."[18]

Lesser efficacy is only one of the reasons that patient advocates lobby not only to win and retain access to whole-plant therapy, but also, and this is important, for patients to be able to grow their own plants. Currently, while medical marijuana is legal in many countries throughout the world, fewer than a handful, including Uruguay, South Africa, and all but two provinces in Canada, allow home cultivation. Additionally, while full medical cannabis is legal in 33 states of the United States, only 16 allow some form of home growing. The Marijuana Policy Project (MPP) states, "Home cultivation is not allowed in Arkansas, Connecticut, Delaware, Florida, Illinois, Maryland, Minnesota, New Hampshire,

New Jersey, New York, Ohio, Pennsylvania or the District of Columbia and a special license is required in New Mexico. In Arizona, Massachusetts, Nevada, and North Dakota, patients can only cultivate in some circumstances, such as if they live a certain distance from the nearest dispensary or if they are granted a waiver for financial hardship."[19] Home cultivation is an important aspect of patients' rights because it allows them legal access to the most effective medicine for their conditions while also eliminating one of the largest barriers to medical marijuana for patients: cost. Because insurance companies will not cover cannabis medicine, even in states where it is legal, costs can be prohibitively high. While treatment with whole-plant extracts is still about three times cheaper than the noncovered costs of pharmaceutical alternatives, treatment can still run upward of $700 a month. Although nonprofit organizations like Jason Cranford's Flowering Hope help by donating medicine to families in need, this option is not available everywhere and is not a long-term solution to the price issue. Cranford understands this, which is why he offers clones of his plants to patients and teaches families how to grow and safely make their own medicine.

One mom who decided to try her hand at home growing to alleviate some of the cost of medication is Barbara Bunker. Barbara's journey toward medical marijuana started six years ago in Austin, Texas. She was elated to find out, on the night of her 18th birthday, that she was pregnant with her first child. She and her boyfriend, Joseph Harris, immediately began planning for the baby and imagining their life as parents. Barbara's pregnancy was healthy and normal, and in August of 2011 she gave birth to Novaleigh Michelle Harris. Novaleigh (also known as Nova or Noni) was a small, quiet baby who slept a lot. Barbara admits now that this should have been a red flag, but she was a young, first-time mom, and she didn't suspect that anything was wrong with her beautiful baby girl. At two months old, Nova received a standard screening/blood test, and the results showed low thyroid hormone. The family was referred to an endocrinologist. When they showed up for the appointment that Friday, the specialist took one look at Barbara and said that her neck looked swollen and that she, too, should get a thyroid test. She said that Barbara had probably passed down her thyroid issue to Nova when she was pregnant and that the baby's levels would normalize over time.

Nova then went in for her MRI, which was supposed to take around

30 minutes. Her parents ended up waiting over two hours in the lobby, so they were a bit concerned. However, Nova was fine when she woke up, and they all went home. The next day, a Saturday, they got a call from the endocrinologist at around 5:00 P.M. Barbara automatically knew something was wrong, since doctors don't generally call with test results on the weekend. The doctor told them to pack their bags and get ready to go to the hospital; the MRI had revealed some alarming news. Baby Novaleigh suffered from schizencephaly, an "extremely rare developmental birth defect characterized by abnormal slits, or clefts, in the cerebral hemispheres of the brain. Babies with clefts in both hemispheres (called bilateral clefts) commonly have developmental delays, delays in speech and language skills, and problems with brain-spinal cord communication."[20]

Nova's case was especially severe—she was missing the right side of her brain and both lobes in the back of her brain. Her optical nerves were severely underdeveloped, meaning that she was legally blind. Additionally, her pituitary gland was so underdeveloped that she had panhypopituitarism; her body was not able to make the hormones essential for human life, including cortisol, thyroid hormone, and growth hormone (which explained her small size).

Children with schizencephaly inevitably end up with seizures, but there is no predicting the severity. Some will only have one seizure from time to time, while others will have almost constant seizures. Nova was not to be one of the lucky ones. She had her first seizure at three months old, while Joseph was giving her a bath (for some reason, children with seizure disorders often have their first seizure triggered by a bath). Her seizures accelerated quickly in both frequency and severity. Barbara and Joseph would spend most of the next two years practically living in Dell Children's Medical Center in Austin, Texas, trying everything they could to get Nova's seizures under control. It was a whirlwind time of specialists and research, tubes and surgeries, and pill after pill, trying to find a solution. While Barbara's voice is generally strong and assertive, belying her young age, she falters when recalling this especially difficult time in their lives. She recalls how the seizures progressed from minor spasms to frightening, almost constant all-over seizures. She would find herself "cradling Nova in my arms sitting on my bed while she shook uncontrollably. Her face in shades of white and grey. Foam coming from her mouth, eyes rolled back, and completely unresponsive." Several times, paramedics had to be rushed in to revive Nova. She always seemed to be on the brink of death.

By the end of those two years, Novaleigh had been tried on all six anti-seizure medications available for a child of her age. Like most children with rare seizure disorders and brain malformations, none of the medications were effective in stopping her seizures. Additionally, all of the strong pharmaceuticals had turned the small child into a zombie. Pictures from the time show an obviously drugged child, her head lolling to the side, eyes almost closed. While Barbara and Joseph had been told that their child would never talk or sit up or walk, they were now beginning to wonder if she had any future at all. At this time, their doctor left and they got a new doctor who advised them to try another surgery—a corpus callosotomy paired with a lesionectomy. The surgeons would split her brain down the middle and take out more of one of her lobes in order to try to stop the seizures. The procedure is a risky one. There is no guarantee that it will help the seizures, and it can even end up making them worse. It can also lead to less functionality or even death. Joseph didn't want to try the surgery, but Barbara reluctantly agreed when the doctor said it was their only hope of stopping the seizures. She went ahead and made an appointment in Houston for a special brain scan to prep Nova for the procedure.

However, even with the plans made, Barbara didn't feel good about the surgery. Nona was already missing almost three-quarters of her brain. How could they take more? And what if she didn't survive the surgery? After much consideration, Barbara changed her mind and decided they should move to Colorado instead. She had known about cannabis's efficacy for pediatric seizures since before Nova was born. However, although it was always in the back of her mind, she didn't think it could really work. In fact, she now recalls, "If I'm being completely honest, I thought the idea of it was crazy. That there's no way that something like this could help my daughter." Yet, the two parents had reached the end of their rope and were willing to move halfway across the country to give it a try. Barbara's family was open to the idea of their moving to try cannabis for their daughter, but Joseph's family did not like the idea at all—they thought of marijuana as a "horrible drug." When the couple told their doctor they were not going to get the surgery but instead were going to move Novaleigh to Colorado to try cannabis, the doctor laughed in their faces. He told them that cannabis would never work for the girl because of the structural problems in her brain and that they were "wasting their time."

Nevertheless, Barbara began to prepare for the move. She and Joseph arranged for doctors in Colorado so that Nova would have no break in care. They put a deposit down on an apartment in Colorado Springs, and in May of 2014 they took their $2,000 in savings and made the move. They couldn't even afford a U-Haul, so they loaded their tiny car with their daughter and as many belongings as they could and drove from Austin to Colorado Springs. When they first got to Colorado, they tried Nova on

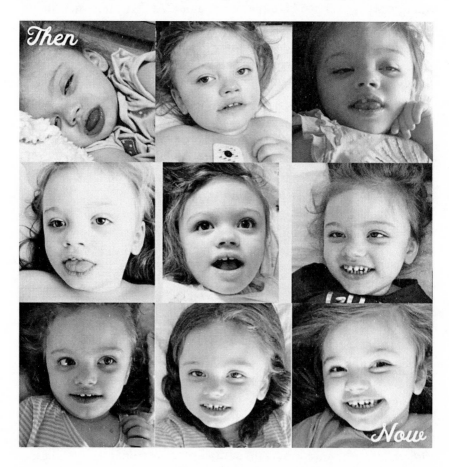

Novaleigh Harris, who has schizencephaly and resultant seizures, shown before and after treatment with cannabis oil (courtesy Barbara Bunker).

CBD oil, since that is the most common cannabis remedy for pediatric seizures. However, not only did the CBD oil not stop her seizures it actually made them worse. They were discouraged but decided not to give up. Some other medical refugees recommended THC oil instead, and they found their "magic bullet." Within weeks, Nova's seizures were reduced by over 90 percent. Barbara was able to start weaning the girl off of her anti-seizure medicines, and without the heavy sedation of the pharmaceuticals her personality began to emerge. When they took her off of Sabil, they realized that the drug was actually causing her blindness. Soon she regained limited vision. Additionally, her body started making hormones again—first growth hormone and then thyroid hormone—and they were able to take her off those medications as well. Her pan-hypothyroidism had gone into remission, and her brain seemed to be healing itself.

Today Nova is not at all the little girl who lies slumped over in her "pre-cannabis" pictures. She laughs and says "mama." She sits up and plays with her toys. She has also gone up to six months with no seizures at all. Her brain and body are healing themselves and developing in ways that her doctors never thought would be possible. As Barbara states, "It's amazing how much this medicine has changed her life." Nova's improvement is without doubt thanks partially to both Colorado's liberal laws surrounding medical marijuana and producers like Jason Cranford developing the most effective strains and products. However, while Barbara and her family have been able to access high-quality oils from the system, money is still tight for the couple, with Colorado's cost of living much higher than in their native Texas. In an informal online poll, medical users in Colorado reported that their monthly cost of cannabis bought from dispensaries ranged from $200-$1,000 a month, depending on the ages and sizes of the patients and their conditions.

Fortunately Barbara has been able to take advantage of Colorado's liberal home-grow laws, an impossibility in so many other medical states. In 2016 she started growing her own plants and with help from the community learned how to make medicine at home for her daughter. The ability to home grow and home produce is a key cost saver, especially for the families of special needs children who spend huge amounts on medical care, caregiving, and special equipment for their kids. It is therefore imperative that medical marijuana laws preserve this right for patients, giving them an alternative to buying from dispensaries or phar-

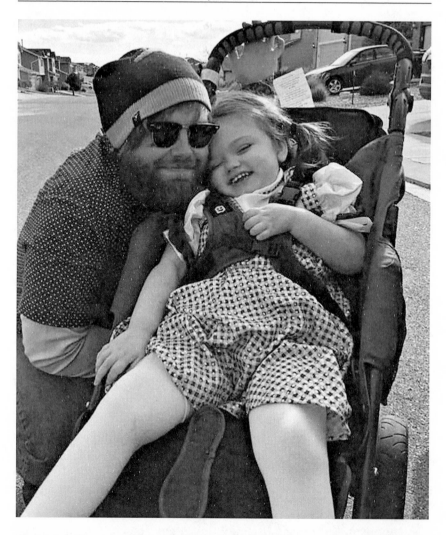

Novaleigh Harris, whose seizures are now well controlled by cannabis, goes trick or treating with her father, Joseph Harris, in Colorado (courtesy Barbara Bunker).

maceutical companies. While cannabis activists around the country continue to fight for regulations in their states that balance the rights of producers and patients, Barbara and Joseph are happy to be living in Colorado, healing Nova in ways they never thought possible. As Barbara says, "My only regret is not coming here sooner."

CHAPTER 4

Refugee Community

Amy Dawn Bourlon-Hilterbran doesn't seem to be your typical organizer or activist. She speaks in a soft Oklahoma accent, and on her Facebook page describes herself as a "small town girl, devoted mother and loving wife." Her friendly soft-spoken manner, however, camouflages a fierce determination. While she has always been active and outgoing, becoming the mother to a special needs child has transformed this mother of eight and grandmother of four into an incredibly effective organizer and activist with an impressive list of accomplishments. She is the founder and CEO of the Millennium Grown Broadcast Network, a medical patients representative and member of the Colorado Health Resource Council, the Colorado State Chair of CannaMoms, and the creator and president at Talk to the 6630507 Hand, a campaign that fights anti-cannabis propaganda. Amy's proudest achievement is the founding of American Medical Refugees (AMR), a network of cannabis patients and families that grew from sharing files on Facebook to the foundation of the medical marijuana community in Colorado. Her LinkedIn profile describes her as a warrior, and indeed she seems to have endless energy in working for medical marijuana patients in Colorado and across the country.

Amy's involvement with the medical cannabis community began, like so many others, when her son Austin started having untreatable seizures. Austin was born in Houston, where Amy had moved with her husband. By the time Austin was born in 2001, she was a single mom raising three kids, so she decided to move back to her hometown of Choctaw, Oklahoma, to be near her family and to start school at the University of Oklahoma. Austin had a few seizures as a baby and toddler, but Amy and others in her family had also had seizures when they were young and had "grown out" of them. Given this family history, doctors were not too worried and assumed that the young boy would stop having seizures just as his mom had. However, between the ages of four and five, Austin's seizures began to go out of control. By this point, Amy had married Jason Hilterbran and was an honors college senior, studying International Area Studies and Political Science. She was very active at the university and in her community despite her one-hour commute to school and the responsibilities of raising three kids. She hoped to work in Africa after completing her degree (she had worked there previously), possibly with the UN, but those plans would soon go out the window.

Within the span of a year, Austin's seizures became unmanageable, even with a plethora of pharmaceuticals. He started to have hundreds of drop seizures every day, and the potent drugs he was on, with their severe side effects, began to take their toll on his physical and mental well-being. The drugs and hospital visits soon put a strain on the family's financial resources as well, and they almost declared bankruptcy before going on Medicare. Jason was working as a firefighter, and, although she was close to completing her degree, Amy had to leave school to stay home and take care of Austin full time. In a story all too familiar among medical marijuana refugees, the family would spend the next four years desperately trying to get Austin's seizures under control. They tried pharmaceutical after pharmaceutical with little result. Eventually Austin could no longer go to school, and his life had been reduced to "literally just lying in his bed sleeping and seizing."

Austin's seizures were so severe that he ended up on life support six times due to seizure activity. The seventh time he ended up on life support was different, however. He was 12 years old, and he was in the hospital on life support because all of the prescription drugs he had been taking daily since the age of four were starting to shut his organs down. At this point, the doctors said that they had done all they could do. Austin was not even a candidate for surgery since the doctors said, "VNS doesn't usually work for Dravet's kids" (VNS surgery is the implantation of a Vagus Nerve Stimulator to try to control seizures). The Hilterbrans had reached the end of the line. Like many parents of critically ill children, Amy had spent years researching independently to try to find a solution for her child. During her time at the University of Oklahoma she had read about some of the research on medical mar-

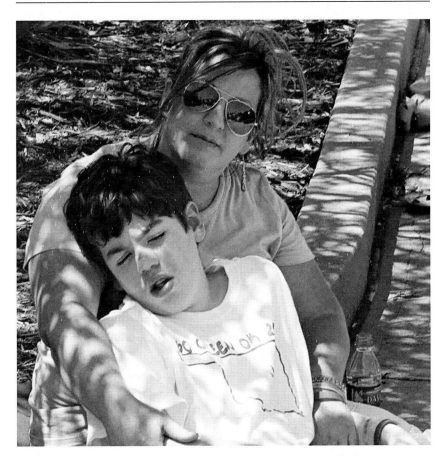

Before treatment with cannabis, Austin Hilterbran was on a plethora of pharmaceuticals, none of which controlled his hundreds of drop seizures a day. Eventually, as his mother, Amy Dawn Bourlon-Hilterbran (pictured here with Austin), recalls, he was just "lying in bed, seizing and sleeping" (courtesy Jason Hilterbran).

ijuana, including Dr. Raphael Mechoulam's groundbreaking studies in Israel. Thus, she was already aware that pediatric epilepsy patients had experienced some relief with CBD oil and other cannabis medications.

The Hilterbrans knew they needed to do something for Austin to try to save his life, and given what Amy had learned about medical marijuana they decided to try cannabis. The couple were not willing to break the law however, so they decided to try to change the law instead. In 2014 they set out to get medical marijuana on the ballot in Oklahoma.

Although polls showed that a majority of the citizens of the state approved of the measure, the regulations in the state are such that it is very difficult for small groups and individuals to get issues on the ballot for general voter approval. The state requires advocates to gather twice as many signatures in half the time of any other state. Amy recounts, "The system is set up to favor big money constituents at the expense of grassroots efforts." Although medical marijuana has since been legalized in Oklahoma, the petition failed in August of that year. By that time Austin was "seizing, seizing, seizing." The family knew they didn't have much time, so they immediately started selling their belongings and getting ready to move to Colorado to try cannabis oil.

Amy and Austin arrived in Colorado Springs in October. Jason stayed in Oklahoma, where he was still working as a firefighter, making the trip back and forth between the two states as often as he could. Amy finally was able to get her son on cannabis oil, within two months of the move. She first started him on THC-A because he was still taking high amounts of benzodiazepine anti-seizure drugs, some of which she had been told could react with CBD oil. THC-A is a cannabinoid found in raw or live cannabis that does not have the psychoactive properties of THC. It has been found to have medicinal value, including anti-inflammatory properties, neuro-protection, and antiemetic properties.[1] The plan was to use THC-A to wean him off his benzodiazepines, particularly a strong version called Onfi (generic name clobazam), which can interact badly with cannabis, then get him started on CBD oil. However, Austin started having "hideous" withdrawals from his pharmaceuticals, making it impossible to focus on anything else. Like many other refugee parents, in the absence of advice from the medical establishment, Amy reached out to other families who were using cannabis oils for their children. She learned from another parent that THC oil could be helpful in abating benzo withdrawal symptoms. She also found out that THC oil rubbed into a child's gums could stop a seizure faster than traditional "rescue" meds. At the time, Austin was using clonazepam to pull out of a seizure, but as a benzodiazepine the medication was rough on him. It took him a long time to recover after each seizure.

With this newfound information, Amy was able to adjust Austin's medicines, and they quickly started to see positive results. She had known the cannabis was working from day one (when they started the

THC-A) because he had no seizures that day, which was unheard of for him. However, she soon saw many improvements beyond seizure reduction. Before he began using cannabis, Austin had clapped his hands as hard as he could repetitively, thousands of times a day for years. After starting cannabis oil, this behavior disappeared. Also, before cannabis, when he was still on multiple pharmaceuticals, he couldn't walk without assistance and could barely stand. He would just lean over and drool. Amy remembers "he was a pharmaceutical zombie." However, after starting cannabis treatment, he was pharmaceutical free within nine months. He now has 95 percent fewer seizures and easily walks without assistance. His life has been completely transformed.

Amy and Jason were thrilled that cannabis had such great results, especially since they weren't sure the plant would help. As Amy says,

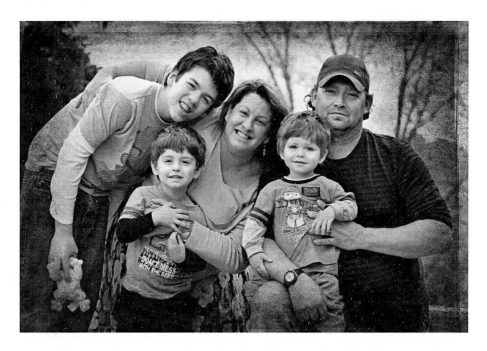

The Hilterbran family (from left: Austin, Nathaniel, Amy, Freeman and Jason). After moving to Colorado and starting on cannabis oil, Austin Hilterbran's seizures were reduced by over 90 percent and he was able to start living a more normal life. Since the move Amy and Jason's younger sons have also had seizures, but early treatment with cannabis has solved the problem (courtesy Nichole Montanez).

they made the move on a "wing and a prayer." Still, the relocation was tough on them. Jason had to stay in Oklahoma for a while because of his job, and after making the move for good he was never able to find another position in firefighting. Additionally, they faced many of the same issues as other patients who relocate for marijuana, including isolation, lack of information, discrimination, and financial struggles. Money can be a huge problem for medical marijuana refugees when they arrive in Colorado. Many families are already financially strained, having spent massive amounts of money on medical care prior to turning to cannabis. Then after leaving jobs and making a costly move they end up in one of the priciest areas of the country.

The cost of living in Colorado as a whole is only slightly higher than the national average, but cannabis patients generally need to be near good medical care and large hospitals, meaning that they need to move to the Denver metro area rather than the cheaper rural areas of the state. Additionally, the Front Range (the eastern slope of the mountains ranging from Fort Collins in the north, through Boulder and Denver, and down to Colorado Springs) tends to be where most job opportunities are. These areas also have incredibly high housing costs. Zillow shows that home prices in Colorado went up 9.8 percent in 2016, giving Colorado some of the most expensive communities in the nation.[2] In Boulder, home prices have grown 308 percent since 1991, over double the national average, making it the number one housing market in the country according to an analysis by SmartAsset. Other Colorado metro areas are growing quickly and getting more expensive as well, with Fort Collins and the Denver Metro area also showing up on the top ten list for growing real estate markets in the country. In 2016 the median single family home price in Boulder rose 14 percent from the previous year, from $790,000 to $905,000. Down the road in the Denver metro area, the single family home median price was a much more reasonable $398,000, while farther south, in Colorado Springs, the median price was an even more affordable $298,000.[3]

While the lower prices of the Colorado Springs area explain why many refugee families settle in that city and surrounding towns, these median costs are still a 13.3 percent increase from the previous year and often much higher than the communities from which families are moving. Unfortunately, rents are even more pricey in regard to national averages. Rents in Colorado as a whole grew at twice the national average between 2015 and 2016, partly due to rising population in the state. Median rent for a two-bedroom apartment was $1,770 in Denver in 2016, with two-bedroom apartments in surrounding suburbs running between $1,300 and $1,700 on average. Again, Colorado Springs proved a much cheaper alternative, with median rent for a two-bedroom apartment running around $1,000. Still, that median price is higher than in many surrounding states, and when you add in Colorado's higher-priced utilities, relocated families often have a hard time.[4]

As if dealing with a higher cost of living weren't bad enough for patients already struggling with medical and financial strains, many families relocating for medical cannabis report discrimination in housing and medical care when they arrive to the state. When Vicki Pletka and her wife, Rosalinda Wirth, moved to Colorado in 2015 to seek treatment with cannabis for their daughter Lily, they traded a three-bedroom house with a large yard in Wisconsin that rented for $750 a month for a small two-bedroom apartment in Colorado Springs that cost $1,100 a month. While at first the apartment seemed fine, they soon realized that the complex had problems with bugs and crime. Then they started being harassed. First their mixed race son was treated poorly by the apartment manager (who didn't believe he lived there) and then they started receiving complaints about Lily, a special needs child, being too loud. Without explanation their lease was not renewed and they had only 30 days to find a new place to live. Other patients have complained about doctors refusing to treat them when they find out they are using cannabis. Some new residents report that they have heard disparaging comments toward refugees, blaming them for Colorado's rising housing costs and increased traffic.

While Amy Dawn Bourlon-Hiltebran and her family also had to deal with financial struggles after their move to Colorado, she found the isolation one of the biggest challenges. Amy and Jason both come from a long line of Oklahoman families. They both graduated from the same high school in Choctaw, where their parents and grandparents were raised. All of their family and friends are in that area, and they thought their kids would go to the same high school as well. When they got to Colorado, they had few contacts—just a couple of other cannabis moms that Amy had friended on Facebook and provider and caretaker

Jason Cranford, who gave them advice even though Austin was not one of his patients. Amy was "appalled" that there was really no cannabis community, and she found it hard to get information in what she describes as a very "dog eat dog" atmosphere. Eventually, she decided to start a Facebook page where people could upload files to share with others who were relocating for cannabis. She called it American Medical Refugees (AMR), and the phrase "medical refugee," which was already being used by a few families who had moved for cannabis, was officially coined.

From the start it was controversial to use a term reserved for international immigrants fleeing political prosecution for those mostly moving from one state to another. In fact, in 2016 the organization briefly considered taking "refugee" out of the name when they were flagged during a fundraising campaign for a food drive. They had a GoFundMe page, but their funds were frozen because of the term "refugee" in their name. They were contacted to ask if they were harboring or aiding Syrian refugees and had to explain that the organization dealt with a different type of "refugee." Amy then talked with a friend in risk management who reassured her, and she decided that medical refugee was the best description. According to the U.S. Department of State, a refugee is "someone who has fled from his or her home country and cannot return because he or she has a well-founded fear of persecution based on religion, race, nationality, political opinion or membership in a particular social group."[5] While this situation is clearly quite different than that faced by medical marijuana refugees, there are also similarities. Medical refugees have to leave their state for fear of persecution if they use the medicine (cannabis) that is most effective for them. Not only could they lose access to a lifesaving medicine but breaking the law in their home state could also result in prosecution, jail time, or the loss of their children, even if they live just miles from the Colorado border.

In April of 2017 one such patient, Larry Burgess, was preparing dinner for his family in Fredonia, Kansas, when his home was surrounded by Wilson County sheriff's deputies with their weapons drawn. Burgess was placed under arrest and had his cannabis medication and related items seized by law officers. Burgess uses cannabis to treat debilitating seizures. At the time of his arrest, he had one plant in his home, as well as some oil extract. His seizures returned quickly after he was taken into custody when he was not able to take his medicine; he had one seizure that night and one the following morning. While Burgess knows that the drug is illegal in Kansas, even for medical use, it is the only remedy that he has found to eliminate his seizures. He and his wife Shannon had been going to Colorado every few months to buy marijuana, but due to rising costs he had decided to start growing his own. The couple also had plans to move to Colorado to access the medicine but needed to wait until their son finished high school. Meanwhile, Burgess faces "six counts, including possession and manufacture of a controlled substance, possession with intent to distribute, and possession of paraphernalia," and has lost all access to the medicine he needs.[6]

The necessity of leaving one's home state was often even more urgent for the first refugees to flee to Colorado, including Sierra Riddle, whose son, Landon, was the first child in America to hold a medical marijuana card. Sierra's battle for Landon to use cannabis would pave the way for those who came later and lay the foundation for the community of medical refugees that exists in Colorado today. While, like many of the refugees that came after her, Sierra had to flee her home state when it became clear that cannabis was the only hope to save her son's life, she also faced challenges in Colorado that, due to ensuing activism and community support, later refugees would not have to confront.

In September of 2012 single mom Sierra Riddle was living in St. George, Utah, with her two-year-old son, Landon. After she noticed that her son had swollen lymph nodes, she took him to the doctor, who diagnosed him with a virus and sent him home. A few days later, however, Sierra noticed that his groin and armpits were also swollen. She took him back to the doctor and received the diagnosis that is a parent's worst nightmare: cancer. Landon was immediately flown to the only pediatric cancer treatment in the state, in Salt Lake City. He was diagnosed with acute lymphocytic leukemia (ALL), a cancer of the blood and bone marrow that is the most common cancer in children. Although the overall survival rate with this form of cancer is around 90 percent, Landon had an extremely aggressive and fast-moving form. By the time he was diagnosed, his mother recalls "his whole chest was full of leukemia tumors."[7] The hospital immediately started treatment but told Sierra that Landon would probably not make it, giving him an 8 percent chance of survival.[8]

Sierra and her mother moved from St. George to Salt Lake City, where Landon would undergo his treatment at a children's hospital. He was scheduled for four years of chemotherapy, along with supplemental radiation therapy. The first year would be inpatient treatment to get rid of the cancer, and the last three years would be treatment at home to maintain remission (what doctors call "consolidation"). Within the first two months of chemotherapy, the doctors saw good progress, as Landon's tumors began to shrink. However, the two-year-old was one of a small percentage of children who could not tolerate the toxic therapy. He would vomit up to 50 times a day and did not eat for over 28 days. Even with IV feeding, he soon dropped from 40 pounds to 20 pounds, literally wasting away. The doctors put him on dozens of strong pharmaceuticals for pain, nausea and anxiety, including Oxycontin, Ativan, morphine, Promethazine and Zofran, to try to ease the side effects of his treatment, but nothing seemed to work. By the end of three months Lan-

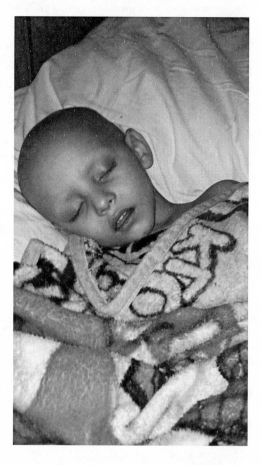

In 2012 Landon Riddle was diagnosed with acute lymphocytic leukemia and given an 8 percent chance of survival. Instead of helping him, conventional chemotherapy and radiation therapy nearly killed him (courtesy Sierra Riddle).

don had lost his ability to walk from neuropathy (nerve damage from his treatments), could no longer talk due to the constant vomiting, and was extremely lethargic. As his mom recalls, "he basically just slept and vomited." The treatment was taking a toll on Landon's mental health too, as he increasingly began to resist his chemotherapy, crying and screaming when nurses tried to administer the pills. He would later tell *Newsweek*, "The chemo actually has healed a lot of kids, but it almost killed me."[9]

Meanwhile, a friend had started a fundraising page for Landon to help with the tens of thousands of dollars of debt they were racking up with his treatments. As people from around the country read about his situation, some began to suggest cannabis, if not to cure his cancer then at least as an aid in dealing with the therapy. At first neither Sierra nor her mom wanted to consider marijuana. But Sierra's mom, despite having been raised with the idea that marijuana is a dangerous drug akin to heroin, began to do some research. Although they could not find any information about children using marijuana for cancer, the word got out, and they were soon contacted by the Stanley brothers from Colorado, who believed they could help the family. The Stanleys actually flew out to Utah to meet with Sierra and her mom and talk about the possibilities of Landon's starting on cannabis.

At around this same time, it became clear that Landon's cancer treatment was killing him. Despite blood and platelet transfusions and dozens of drugs, as his mother says "the chemo was shutting his body down." The hospital decided to give him a two-week "break" from the chemo, saying that they would restart the therapy when, and if, his body rebounded. They also were going to provide him with a home hospice nurse, a frightening sign that they didn't expect him to survive. Sierra and her mom picked up Landon from the hospital and drove to the pharmacy to pick up the medications and IVs they would need for the two-week stint, but then instead of driving to their temporary Salt Lake City home they headed over the snow-covered mountains and down to Colorado Springs. They were going to give cannabis a try.

The Riddles stayed with Joel and Amanda Stanley, and Landon took his first cannabis dose (a special THC/CBD strain the Stanleys had been breeding) on January 22, 2013. Sierra recalls that "it was amazing to see how well he did, even just after that first dose." Landon's condition continued to improve over those next two weeks, and the Riddles knew that cannabis would now be part of Landon's treatment. They could not move at that point, though, so they decided to take up dual residency, finishing Landon's last year of chemo in Salt Lake City but travelling back and forth to Colorado Springs (where the Stanleys had set up a room in their own house for them) so that Landon could continue taking cannabis. All of this was happening at around the same time Charlotte Figi was receiving treatment for her epilepsy from the Stanleys. The media soon took notice. Landon was also filmed by CNN for Sanjay Gupta's *Weed* special at the same time as Charlotte, although his footage was not used initially since he was taking THC. While Charlotte was using the special high–CBD strain that was named for her, Landon was taking high doses of CBD and THC (500 mg a day of CBD and 1,000 mg per day of THC), and because of THC's psychoactive properties his doses were much more controversial. Still, Gupta did eventually air the footage of Landon, and the Riddles were forced to leave Utah the very next day or face prosecution in that state.

By this time, Landon had been in chemotherapy for a year and his cancer was in remission. The doctors in Salt Lake City were amazed by his progress and essentially encouraged Sierra to continue cannabis therapy. She remembers the oncologist saying to her on the day of Landon's discharge, "Honestly Sierra, I have treated a lot of children with leukemia, and I did not think that Landon would survive.... [W]hatever you are doing, keep doing it, don't stop." So the Riddles packed up and moved to Colorado Springs, where they thought the worst would be behind them. Sierra had recently been certified as a nursing assistant so she could care for Landon at home. She decided that since he was in remission, and since treatment was so hard on him, they would forego the three more years of chemotherapy and just treat with cannabis. She headed to Children's Hospital with Landon's transfer papers to find a new oncologist, and, as she says, "that is when our nightmare began."

The Denver oncologist did not agree with Sierra's foregoing the rest of Landon's chemotherapy in favor of cannabis treatment. In fact, she said that if Sierra did not agree to the conventional treatment plan, the hospital would call child protective services (CPS) on her. And that is exactly what happened. CPS was waiting for Sierra when she got home from that appointment. The Riddles would spend the next 18 months fighting the medical establishment to treat Landon in the way they felt was best. The Children's Hospital team called CPS on Sierra a dozen times, and she could not find any doctors in the state to back her up, including the MD who had originally signed Landon's medical card. Because he was the youngest patient in the state at the time, no doctors were willing to possibly lose their licenses to recommend cannabis over chemotherapy. But Sierra knew that her son was healthy now and refused to put him through three more years of the therapy that almost killed him. She brought a lawsuit against the hospital and was eventually able to find doctors and researchers from out of state to back her position.

The Riddles and the hospital finally came to an agreement that the doctors would do a bone marrow aspiration, a spinal tap and blood tests. If they found any cancer cells, Landon would restart chemotherapy; however, if Landon was cancer free they would remove his chemo port and that would be the end of it. Fortunately Landon was 100 percent cancer free, and the port was removed from his chest the following week. Sierra never heard from that oncologist again. In 2018 Landon turned nine and celebrated six years of being cancer free. He continues cannabis treatment to deal with the damage done from the chemo and radiation therapy. His neuropathy is now gone and he has started to catch up in his growth. However, he has dental damage from chemotherapy and brain damage from the cranial radiation, which has slowed his learning. He also suffers from PTSD due to the trauma he endured at such a young age, but ongoing cannabis therapy helps with that. Despite these continuing issues from his conventional treatment, Sierra knows she made the right decision to

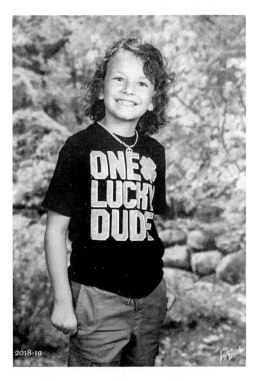

After moving to Colorado and being treated with cannabis oil, Landon Riddle's cancer went into remission. Here he is, healthy and happy, in his 2018–2019 school photograph (courtesy LifeTouch Photography).

move to Colorado and fight for Landon to use cannabis. Today he is a healthy, happy kid who is in school and doing "so, so well."

Sierra's bravery in moving states and standing down the medical establishment has had repercussions far beyond her son's health. Children's Hospital has since changed its pediatric oncology team and its policies on cannabis treatment. In fact, one of their MDs, Dr. Nick Foreman, is currently leading research on cannabis and pediatric cancer. Additionally, Sierra gets thousands of e-mails, calls, and messages every month from parents who want information about marijuana and pediatric cancer. Because she was willing to stand up for her son and go to the media with her story, many parents have learned about cannabis treatment. She is a true pioneer in the cannabis community in Colorado, and her bravery has paved the way for the formation of the thriving medical refugee community that exists today.

Sierra Riddle is an exemplar for the thousands of patients who are forced to move from their states or face arrest. In addition, like other medical refugees, she cannot return to her home state of Utah to visit family for fear of prosecution if Landon tests positive for THC.[10] This is a common complaint of medical refugees, who not only have to move away from their home state but are also then "captive" in their new state because they cannot legally travel with their medicine. As mentioned previously, crossing state lines with marijuana, even between two legal states, falls under federal jurisdiction. The federal government considers taking any Schedule I drug from one state to another to be drug trafficking, a felony offense.[11] Yes, medical refugees are usually U.S. citizens who have the freedom to move to another state and can speak the local language, but they still face legal and health risks if they do not move to legally access their medicines or if they do not stay in their new, legal state. There are other similarities between international refugees and medical refugees. Medical refugees usually have to leave friends and family behind, sometimes for good. They have to quit their jobs, sell or give away their belongings, and often end up in extreme financial hardship. And while they do know the culture and language of their new community they still are often alone, and they have the added hardship of chronic or terminal illnesses. So, like international refugees, medical refugees tend to move to areas with particular characteristics, one of the most important being an existing community of other refugees.

The importance of community has been clearly demonstrated by those who study international refugees. The United States has resettled over three million international refugees since the Refugee Act of 1980. And while refugees have settled in all 50 states, they do tend to move to particular areas; for example, in 2016 California, New York, and Texas settled almost a quarter of all refugees.[12] Many factors determine where refugees are settled, but the most important are volunteer or church organizations in the area, a welcoming local community and economic opportunities. Refugees themselves can also request to resettle where they already have family or know of other refugees from the same country or culture. This last fact can explain why certain cities become havens for refugees from particular regions. Minneapolis, for example, is "home to a large Somali population that settled in the early 1990s during the Somali civil war."[13] Smaller cities can also become destinations for refugees. Lancaster, Pennsylvania (population 59,302), has settled over 1,300 refugees from the Middle East since 2013, earning it the nickname of "America's Refugee Capital." While this is partly because of two religious nonprofits, Church World Services and Bethany Christian Services, it is also due to a welcoming local attitude and a growing community of refugees from similar cultures.[14]

In Colorado there are also communities of international refugees, with the suburban community of Aurora, just outside of Denver, one of the largest. Almost all international refugees that come to Colorado end up in Aurora, where one in five residents is foreign born. The *Denver Post* notes, "The Ethiopian community alone in the Aurora-Denver area in the eastern part of the metro area is an estimated 30,000 strong. Part of that number includes refugees."[15] Several factors contribute to Aurora's large refugee community, including cheap rent and a community of international refugees already in place. The city also has a refugee clinic, welcome centers for refugees in public schools, and the Immigrant and Refugee Commission.[16] All of these aspects are important in attracting and creating a livable community for refugees.

Amy Dawn Bourlon-Hiltebran felt the need for a similar type of community for medical marijuana refugees when she first started the AMR Facebook page in 2015. The group grew quickly as people joined the page and shared files on doctors, housing, oil doses, etc. However, although it was now easier for patients to get and share information,

Amy still felt isolated and yearned for some face-to-face community. Easter was approaching, a time she would usually be spending with extended family back in Oklahoma. She figured that many other relocated families would be feeling the same way, so she decided to organize an Easter egg hunt in nearby Cañon City, Colorado. She publicized the event on the Facebook page and was shocked when over 150 people showed up. The medical refugee community was out there; it was just that nobody had organized them before.

At this point Amy realized the great need for community among the cannabis refugees, and she decided to expand the Facebook page to a real organization with events and get-togethers. She decided to focus primarily on holiday events, since that tends to be the most isolating time for patients who are far away from family and friends and who generally cannot travel. Since that time, AMR has hosted events for Mother's Day, Father's Day, July 4, Halloween, and more. They have organized refugee family days at local baseball games and have had potlucks, fundraisers and donation drives in various locales throughout the state. Currently they host four events every month, including potlucks and book groups in both Colorado Springs and Denver, as well as events for every major holiday, along with food drives and other giveaways. The incredible growth of the organization in just a few years shows not only the growing medical marijuana refugee population in Colorado but also the need for an organized support system for that community.

In 2017, with membership having grown to over 230 families, AMR became an official nonprofit, changed its name to American Medical Refugee Foundation, and filed for 501c3 status. According to Amy, it was important for the organization to take the next step in order to better serve the growing number of refugee families in Colorado. With nonprofit status, the foundation will be more effectively able to raise funds, which will help not only to pay for special events but also to set up a grant program to help new families with expenses. Additionally, the Hilterbrans realized that while helping out cannabis families will always be a key component of the organization it was also necessary to push for education and political change. Amy says, "There isn't room for every medical cannabis user in Colorado, even if they want to move here." One of AMR's commitments is to challenge marijuana refugees to stay politically aware in their hometowns, states, and countries so that they can make needed change there. To that end, the foundation has opened chapters in prohibition states like Texas to help families push for medical marijuana reform in their own states.

In addition to community support and political activism, part of AMR's mission is education, and the group holds seminars and workshops on a variety of topics such as making one's own medical oils. However, Amy realized soon after starting the group that more needed to be done to inform the greater public about medical marijuana and that she was going to need to start a business that could also help to provide for her family's financial needs. By this time, the family was living in Florence, Colorado (a less expensive small town near Colorado Springs), and her husband was working as a contractor. However, they now had two more small children and money was tight. So in the summer of 2015 Amy and her husband decided to start a media network based on cannabis issues—Millennium Grown Broadcast Network. Amy had previously worked in sales and marketing for media and was aware of the inter-workings of media networks. She decided that MGB would have a variety of shows catering to different aspects of the audience, including a veterans' show, a women's hour, a teen medical use show, and others. Currently the network broadcasts on Blog Talk Radio, features a YouTube channel, and has other live-stream broadcasts on cannabis topics. Additionally, the network hosts a monthly VIP gathering of cannabis industry insiders with talks by experts and fundraising for the American Medical Refugees Foundation.

Both American Medical Refugees and Millennium Grown Broadcast Network have helped to bring the cannabis community together in Colorado, providing support and information while being joined by other groups such as CannaMoms, Weed for Warriors, and Cannabis Patients Alliance. Unfortunately, as a high-profile group of refugee families, the organization has sometimes served as a target for the same sort of scam artists who have ripped off individual refugees in apartment leases or cannabis-oil services. The vulnerability of families dealing with very ill children while living in new areas where they know few people can attract hucksters looking to make easy money. Amy says, "Desperate people do desperate things, and by design every refugee is desperate. They are fighting daily to save someone they love, and that is the most vulnerable person on the planet." So when someone says "this medicine will help your child—give me your money," they are ready to bite. She continues: "We are just fish in a pond, and there are more and more fish every day."

One of the first scams that the group had to deal with involved a man who infiltrated the group, saying that he had epilepsy and experience working with special needs children. He was very friendly and seemed knowledgeable, so when he contacted a member about helping her with her child's IEP (Individualized Education Program, a written plan that is developed for each public school student who is eligible for special education) in exchange for room and board, she accepted the offer. He said he had done this work all over the country and was an expert at representing parents to schools for writing IEPs. However, when the single mom approached the school district and told them he would be representing the member, they warned her that he sounded very similar to a man they had heard about. They described a man who was a scam artist and pretended to be an expert on IEPs, then approached single mothers with special needs kids and later stole from them. The mom checked into it and, in fact, it was the same man. He had previously been working an identical hoax with parents in an autistic kids' group in Texas, and he even had an FBI file for fraud. Unfortunately, at this point he was already on a bus heading to the member's home in Colorado. She quickly informed AMR, and they convened a group of members to meet him at the bus station and inform him that they knew who he was and had called the police. He quickly left Colorado but has since moved on to other states and even other countries, where he works the same type of fraud on vulnerable, unsuspecting parents.

This scam not only reflects the vulnerability of medical refugees but also the fledgling cannabis industry and the greed of some unscrupulous people who try to make money off of medical misfortune and desperation. Amy and other refugees have dozens of stories of fraudulent products and "experts" who were anything but. In 2015 a man joined AMR under the pretense of being a medical refugee from Louisiana with IBS and other digestive issues. He posted on the page and even came to events, where he availed himself of free food and product giveaways. Meanwhile, he was gathering information from the multiple files on AMR's page—information that Amy had spent years compiling for the benefit of other refugees. He then started the Cannabis Consulting Company and charged people for the information he had taken from AMR's page. The pain is evident in Amy's voice when she talks about the experience. For the first few years, Amy and her husband funded AMR from their own pocket. They genuinely want to help others in the community, and while they have since started screening members more carefully it will always be impossible to keep out every unethical individual.

Despite these setbacks, Amy's organizational and networking skills have been key in bringing together a previously disjointed group of people into a community and providing support, information, and friendship to medical refugees. In fact, many of the refugees I spoke with told me that AMR was a decisive factor in their choice to move to Colorado and to settle in the Colorado Springs area, where over half of AMR's member families live. The Sanchez family, originally from Texas, decided to move to the Springs in large part because of Amy and AMR. Like most other refugees, the Sanchezes felt nothing but frustration with doctors and hospitals before deciding to move to Colorado to try cannabis. Unlike most other families, however, the Sanchez family was seeking treatment for four of their five family members, all of whom suffer from a rare condition called Glycogen Storage Disease.

Glycogen Storage Disease (GSD) is an "inherited genetic disorder which causes the deficiency of one of the enzymes that work to help the body break down the storage form of sugar (glycogen) into glucose, which the body uses to keep blood sugar stable when a person is not eating."[17] When a person eats, excess glucose is stored in the liver as glycogen, which is then released into the bloodstream as needed to maintain a steady blood sugar level. People with GSD, however, lack the enzyme that converts glycogen to glucose and cannot maintain blood sugar levels. Thus they end up with hypoglycemia (low blood sugar) within a couple of hours of eating. These chronically low blood sugar levels lead to hunger, fatigue, and irritability. Over time, glucose builds up in the patient's liver, causing it to swell. The kidneys can also become enlarged from this disorder. Currently there are no treatments for GSD besides diet. Because of liver involvement, those who suffer from Glycogen Storage Disorder are contraindicated from taking pharmaceutical medications.[18]

While most children are diagnosed with GSD between four and ten months of age, Amanda and Steve Sanchez's oldest daughter, Madison, was not diagnosed until the age of four years. Because it is a rare disease it is often relatively unknown outside of major urban areas (it is more common in the Jewish community and in the northeast United States). Thus it can often be misdiagnosed. Steve also has GSD that was not diagnosed until he was an adult, as does his mother, who was misdiagnosed with diabetes for years. At the time of Madison's diagnosis, Steve and Amanda were living in Corpus Christi, Texas, Steve's hometown. They first took Madison to the local children's hospital because she was having stomach pain and was not gaining weight. The hospital did not really have the ability to diagnose her properly, and, in fact, blamed the family for her small size, saying they were not "feeding her."

The Sanchez family persisted in their efforts to get Madison medical help, however, and were eventually referred to an endocrinologist. The specialist suggested she could have Glycogen Storage Disorder, which was confirmed through special blood tests. The doctor then did an ultrasound and found that, indeed, her liver was extremely swollen. Unfortunately, the doctors were unaware of the proper treatment protocol for GSD and told the family that they needed to feed Madison more sugar to bring up her blood sugar levels. This is actually the opposite of the proper treatment for the disease, however, and Madison's condition did not improve. Steve did some research online and found a GSD specialist in Florida named David Weinstein. Dr. Weinstein was able to confirm Madison's GSD diagnosis and give them the correct treatment protocol, which includes eliminating all sugar from the diet and eating starch every two hours to help the body metabolize properly. Eventually Madison had genetic testing that would confirm she had an extremely rare form of Glycogen Storage Disease. While most people with the disease have a break on one DNA branch, Madison's test showed a break in three different genes. Currently there are only three other people known to have that same genetic anomaly.

After finding out that Madison had Glycogen Storage Disease and that it is inherited, it didn't take long for Steve to find out that he also suffered from the disorder. Additionally, the Sanchezes' younger son, Aaron, who was two at the time, was having trouble sleeping, so they decided to have his blood sugar tested as well. He was soon diagnosed with the disease, and because low blood sugar can cause nocturnal seizures they now had an explanation for his sleepless nights. Soon Aaron was also diagnosed with autism. Doctors wanted to start him on medication for that, but because of GSD and its effects on the liver he was not able to start any pharmaceuticals. Meanwhile, although having a diagnosis for their children (and for Steve) was encouraging, all three family members continued to suffer with symptoms of GSD, including unstable blood sugar. Around this time, Amanda gave birth to their third child, Rize, whose small size and slow growth led them to believe that he, too, had GSD.

The Sanchez family had been battling what they perceived as a "horrible medical system" in Texas for years. In addition to their problems in getting a correct diagnosis for their daughter, Amanda had suffered a botched gall bladder surgery in Corpus Christi a couple of years earlier in which the surgeon cut the wrong bile duct and also nicked her liver, causing her to almost bleed out. Although they were eventually referred to doctors in Houston for the GSD, the Sanchezes didn't find many more answers there. So, early on, they began considering other options. Steve was doing extensive research online and soon came across some research on using cannabis oil to regulate blood sugar. One study, published in the *American Journal of Medicine* in 2013, showed that cannabis compounds may help control blood sugar. The lead researcher, Murray Mittleman from Harvard Medical School, made this statement to *Time*: "The most important finding is that current users of marijuana appeared to have better carbohydrate metabolism than non-users. Their fasting insulin levels were lower, and they appeared to be less resistant to the insulin produced by their body to maintain a normal blood-sugar level."[19] In his online research, Steve also saw information on cannabis repairing damaged DNA, and that was all it took. He knew that they needed to try cannabis oil for their son Aaron, and possibly for other members of the family as well. They first started Aaron on CBD while they were still in Texas. Although CBD is technically legal there, the law is a bit of a grey area so they were still nervous about it. Additionally, they really wanted to try whole-plant oil with THC, so they decided to leave the state in order to be able to treat their children legally.

Steve names one main factor in their decision to choose Colorado over another legal state: "the American Medical Refugees Facebook page." While he had been to Colorado before and knew it was a beautiful state with laid-back attitudes, it was the proof and hope that they saw in the stories on AMR's page that really gave them the push to make the move to the state. In early 2016 they sold almost everything they owed, Steve left the job he had been at for 13 years, and they packed their car and drove to Colorado. They had an apartment lined up in Aurora, close to Children's Hospital, but they soon found out that Colorado Springs was cheaper and had a larger medical refugee community, so like many others they ended up in the Springs. They wasted no time in getting their middle son, Aaron, on cannabis oil, and they began to see results right away. His seizures disappeared and he started sleeping through the night. In fact, he has had only one seizure since the family moved to Colorado, and Amanda believes that it is because she once let up on the cannabis oil a bit.

With Aaron's success, they decided to start Madison on the oil to try to help with the nausea, vomiting, and pain that comes along with Glycogen Storage Disease. She, too, saw dramatic results. When their youngest son, Rize, was eventually diagnosed with GSD, he was also started on the oil. Now all three children have their red cards and are on 1:1 CBD/THC cannabis oil, along with a special diet. They remain symptom free. Steve is also taking cannabis oil for his GSD symptoms. Neither parent has any regrets about uprooting their family and making the move to Colorado. Like most other refugees, they mention that the hardest part of the move was leaving family behind in Texas. This was made even harder by the fact that many of their family members and friends didn't really understand what they were doing. Because GSD is a rare disorder with few outward symptoms, Steve says that many people don't understand how hard living with the disease is. Additionally, their friends and families "didn't understand cannabis" or think it would help the children.

Despite the pushback from their loved ones, the Sanchezes' move was in many ways easier than that of other refugees, in large part due to the community built by American Medical Refugees. Immediately after the move the family went to a Mother's Day event sponsored by AMR. They met many "families and nice people" who would become part of their new "cannabis community" in Colorado. They were able to get their oils at first from Jason Cranford's Flowering Hope Foundation, easing the financial burden, and they are now "sponsored" by another cannabis company, "incredibles." Because of the hard work of those who came before them and a good dose of luck, the Sanchezes were able to make a difficult transition with relative ease, and the whole family is doing better because of it. In fact, while many refugees say they would return to their home states if marijuana were legalized there, Steve and Amanda are happy to stay in Colorado. Steve says, "If they legalized in Texas, even if they were giving it away for free, I would not go back!" The community that has been created by and for refugees in Colorado has helped thousands of patients like the Sanchez family to call Colorado home.

CHAPTER 5

Where's the Research?

In 2015, while refugees were flocking to Colorado to seek treatment for everything from autism to epilepsy, 7,500 miles away a very different story was unfolding. On July 1, 2015, 19-year-old Alex Renton died in his hospital bed in Wellington, New Zealand, surrounded by his family and loved ones. Alex, who was once a "strapping, healthy rugby player," had been in the hospital for three months after he went into status epilepticus for no apparent reason (status epilepticus, or SE, is defined by the Epilepsy Foundation as a seizure that lasts more than five minutes, which, if it cannot be stopped, usually results in death). When the hospital was unable to stop Alex's seizures with conventional antiepileptic drugs, they induced a coma to give his brain a rest. Meanwhile, Alex's mom, Rose, who was aware of the success that seizure patients in the United States were having with cannabis, petitioned the New Zealand Ministry of Health to allow her son access to a CBD-only version of the drug.[1]

Since 2008 chronically or terminally ill patients in New Zealand have been able to apply to the government to use one of two approved CBD-only products—Sativex or Tilray. However, up until 2015 only 59 patients had been approved to use one of the drugs. Partly due to the extremely high costs of these pharmaceuticals (around $875 a month for Sativex, a bit less for Tilray), most marijuana patients in New Zealand reported using cannabis illegally, growing and making their own product.[2] Due to the high cost and low availability of other options, Rose Renton was asking to use another CBD product, Elixinol, which she had been able to acquire from Colorado. After two months of petitioning, Associate Health Minister Peter Dunne gave a one-off approval for the Rentons to use Elixinol on "compassionate grounds," the first ever approval for a "non-pharmaceutical grade product," and the first approval for the use of cannabis in a hospital in New Zealand.[3]

Alex Renton got his first dose of CBD oil on June 16, 2015. His other medications were gradually reduced, he regained consciousness, and his seizures stopped within that first week. By the next week, his mother wrote, "Alex is holding his own and maintaining his own breathing!"[4] Unfortunately, the seizures and months of heavy sedation had taken their toll on Alex's body, and two days later he passed away. While the doctors at the Wellington hospital released a report that the cannabis had made no difference in his condition, his mother was quick to refute their account. She asserted that cannabis did have a role to play but it was given too late and only "after a long battle with medical staff for backing, and after 43 other drugs had failed."[5] And even though the drug did not save her son's life, Rose maintained that it helped to ease his passing, stating that he "died peacefully without heavily layered drugs." In fact, even the hospital admitted that the drug has a "role, particularly in the palliative role—in the dying stage."[6]

While we cannot know for sure if Alex would have lived had he been given cannabis oil at an earlier stage of his illness or if he had gained access to other types of cannabis treatment, individual cases in the United States as well as international studies indicate that the answer could be "yes." International cooperation in regard to both research and policy is clearly a necessity for patients who could benefit from cannabis treatments—in New Zealand, in Colorado, and globally. Although Colorado is currently one of the leaders in medical cannabis policy and countries like Israel lead the way in medical marijuana research, this progress must be shared throughout the world.

In the meantime, back in New Zealand, Rose Renton refuses to let her son's death be in vain. She continues to fight for the rights of ill New Zealanders to access cannabis medicines. In 2016 she created a petition to the House of Representatives asking for easier access to good-quality, affordable medical marijuana.[7] She presented the petition, with 15,000 signatures, to the parliament in October of that year.[8] Apparently such pressure has had an effect, because in June 2017 the government announced that CBD would no longer be classed as a controlled drug, meaning that doctors could prescribe the substance and patients would no longer have to petition the ministry of health to be able to use it.

While this is a step forward for New Zealand, the new policy applies only to CBD products, not any whole-plant or THC medicines. Additionally, with a "limited range of medical-grade CBD products" available in the country, the announcement does not necessarily address issues of cost and access for patients in need.[9] Until patients in New Zealand have laws and distribution systems similar to those in Colorado, patients will continue to suffer needlessly or, in worst-case scenarios, die.

As Alex Renton's situation makes clear, it is not only patients in the U.S. who could benefit from cannabis as medicine. Although there are no statistics on where medical refugees are coming from, a report in the *Guardian* states that a handful of patients are relocating to states like Colorado from other countries including Spain, Ireland, and Germany.[10] This is because Colorado has been a groundbreaker in terms of domestic cannabis policy, and the state is also an exception on an international scale. Currently cannabis is fully legal in only two countries, Uruguay and Canada. Many other countries, including the Netherlands, Mexico, Chile, Costa Rica, and Portugal have decriminalized marijuana, meaning that possession of small amounts is legal but the sale or production of the drug is illegal. Some countries, like Spain and South Africa, have laws that essentially show cannabis as being legal for private consumption but are not considered to have full legalization. Finally, several other countries have legal marijuana for medical purposes only, including Israel, Turkey, Poland, Australia, and, most recently, Germany. Unfortunately, aside from Israel none of these countries has a well-developed medical cannabis system, meaning that they lack medical experts, distribution systems, and other facets important to a medical marijuana program.[11]

With full-spectrum medical marijuana currently legal in 33 states in the U.S., it is clear that the United States is, in some ways, leading the world in cannabis policy. Ironically, it is also the United States that is largely responsible for the prohibition of cannabis on a global scale. Journalist Christopher Moraff has written as follows: "For the past half century, nearly every escalation in the global war on illicit drugs has been reactionary in nature and initiated almost exclusively under U.S. guidance."[12] The world's first drug control treaty came out of the First International Opium Conference in 1912, a 13-nation conference convened by the U.S. The "International Opium Convention" was signed at The Hague that year by Germany, the U.S., China, France, the UK, Japan, Italy, the Netherlands, Persia, Siam, Portugal, and Russia.[13] During the convention these countries pledged to give their "best endeavors" to control and eradicate the opium trade. The convention went into force globally when it was implemented as part of the Treaty of Versailles in 1919.[14] While the first convention applied only to opium, a revised convention, signed in Geneva in 1925, included "Indian Hemp" (as mentioned earlier, "Indian Hemp" was a name used widely for cannabis prior to the 1930s prohibition movement, which favored the name "marijuana").[15] The 1920s was a time during which anti-marijuana propaganda and sentiment was growing in the United States, so it is no surprise that the American delegates pushed for the inclusion of cannabis in the treaty. Marijuana would not be nationally prohibited in the U.S. until the Marihuana Tax Act of 1937, although individual states were outlawing the drug throughout the twenties and early thirties.[16] Of significance was that the revised Opium Convention still allowed the use of "Indian Hemp" "exclusively for medical or scientific purposes."[17]

It wasn't until 1961 that U.S. prohibitionist policies were adopted in the United Nations when the original 73 delegates to the Single Convention on Narcotic Drugs met in New York to create a "global framework" for battling narcotic drugs.[18] One of the architects of this convention was the Narcotics Bureau chief, Harry Anslinger, the man who was almost single-handedly responsible for the nearly century-long war against cannabis in the United States. Ten years later, in 1971, the UN ratified another drug treaty, this time targeting psychotropic substances. It is certainly no coincidence that this was also the year President Richard Nixon launched the modern war on drugs, calling drugs "America's public enemy number 1."[19]

Since that time, the International Narcotics Control Board (INCB), which oversees implementation of the UN's drug control treaties, has stayed firmly in line with the United States' federal prohibitionist policies, including those on marijuana. Despite scientific research, the INCB has questioned the efficacy of smoked marijuana and has criticized Uruguay, Washington state, and Colorado for lifting marijuana prohibitions.[20] Despite the long history of United States influence over the UN's, and subsequently the world's, marijuana policies, the World Health Organization (WHO) met in 2016 to initiate the first steps in a long process that could result in the rescheduling of medical marijuana at the global level. The Expert Committee of Drug Dependence (ECDD), which is part of WHO, makes recommendations to the secretary general of the United Nations, who can then bring the recommendations for a vote by the United Nations Committee on Narcotic Drugs (CND). If the CND approves the recommendations, the recommendations are then voted on by the UN General Assembly. A vote for rescheduling could "result in fundamental changes in the way medical marijuana research and regulations are handled in the United States and around the world."[21]

While change does appear to be on the horizon it is a slow process and may prove too late for many patients, like Alex Renton, who could benefit from medical marijuana on a global level. Many individual countries remain hesitant to go against UN (and U.S.) prohibitionist practices. The Rentons' home country of New Zealand, for example, remains firmly entrenched under U.S. influence in the realm of marijuana policy. In March 2017 I spoke with Chris Fowlie, the president of that country's National Organization for the Reform of Marijuana Laws (NORML), and he explained the power of international treaties and U.S. influence in keeping medical marijuana essentially illegal in their country. Fowlie, who has been involved in marijuana advocacy for 25 years, said that New Zealand is a "small country that must follow treaties." However, he also stated that legalization in the States and elsewhere (like Uruguay and Canada) has definitely helped New Zealand's movement, and they hope to use these places as a template for their own policies. So, even in a country that is 7,500 miles away and across the Pacific Ocean, Colorado's marijuana policies have influence. However, federal legalization and changes to international treaties would be even more effective. Fowlie states, "We're part of a worldwide tide, but we really need U.S. leadership on this." And that leadership needs to be not just in policy but also in scientific research.

Strict prohibitionist policies not only affect the ability of patients to access the drug but also hamper clinical research. One country that has remained at the head of the curve when it comes to research on medical cannabis is Israel. Since Israeli scientist Raphael Mechoulam's discovery of THC at Hebrew University in Jerusalem in 1964, Israeli scientists have continued to lead the way in medical marijuana research, assisted by their country's policies. Medical marijuana has been permitted in Israel since the early 1990s for conditions including cancer, Parkinson's disease, Crohn's disease, multiple sclerosis, chronic pain, and post-traumatic stress disorder. About 25,000 Israelis, out of a population of 8.5 million, use medical cannabis,[22] a number sure to grow as the industry expands in that country. Israel is one of only three countries in the world that provide government-grown cannabis to medical patients, and it currently has multiple grow operations. "Breath of Life will soon open a 1-million-square-foot grow-house and research center in southern Israel. The space will be among the largest medical cannabis growth and R&D facilities in the world, according to Viridian Capital Advisors, a financial firm focused on the cannabis market."[23]

This consistent source of quality medicine also helps Israel remain the leader in clinical research on the drug. Its health ministry currently funds dozens of trials and has written protocols on the matter known as the "Green Book." Dr. Mechoulam, the scientist who discovered THC, remains involved in cannabis research in Israel, as well as collaborating with researchers around the world. He told the *New York Times* in December 2016 "medicinal cannabis has to follow medical lines of thought and development and modern medical routes." He is also surprised by the lack of clinical trials at the international level, stating, "Israel has more than the United States at the moment, which is ridiculous."[24] With its investment in research and medicine, Israel stands poised to lead the industry as cannabis medicines become more widely accepted in the years ahead.

Meanwhile, in the United States doctors and scientists struggle to carry out medical marijuana research due to federal limitations, even in states like Colorado. Dr. Alan Shackelford is a Denver-based physician who specializes in behavioral and occupational health but is also a medical marijuana doctor and advocate. He first became frustrated with the lack of information and research about cannabis in the U.S. around 2009, when patients he was treating for chronic pain began to ask him about medical marijuana. He was trying to figure out dosage, how to administer the drug, etc., but found relatively few research studies. After locating a couple of studies, including one from Washington State University published that year on the uses of medical marijuana, he decided to go ahead and use the drug with his patients, especially those with pain who did not respond to conventional treatments with narcotics. As he continued to look into the research and saw his patients responding positively to the drug, he became "more and more interested in it" and soon switched his focus from occupational medicine to marijuana. However, despite his long and storied career in medicine, including appointments at New England Deaconess and Harvard Medical School, Dr. Shackelford still had to teach himself about cannabis. Every year, he discovered more and more research, including a 2010 paper on using marijuana to treat neuropathic pain by Marc Wehr from McGill University, and a 2011 paper on the same topic by Donald Abrams from the University of California at San Francisco. Dr. Shackleford was reassured to see his observations being upheld by studies, and he began to recommend marijuana not only for pain but also for cancer, muscle spasms, and glaucoma.

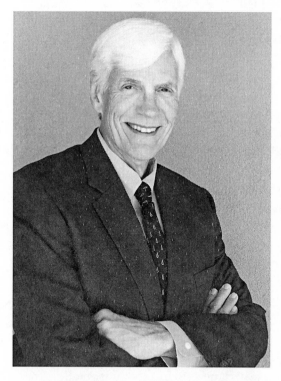

Dr. Alan Shackelford, MD, was the first doctor in Colorado to recommend cannabis for a pediatric patient. He continues to be at the forefront of medical marijuana research (courtesy Vanessa Reich-Shackelford).

All was going smoothly until he was approached by Charlotte Figi, the five-year-old Dravet's patient, and her mother in 2012. Much as he had been initially hesitant to treat pain with cannabis due to his lack of familiarity with the drug, he was now hesitant to treat a child with the substance since he did not have any knowledge of its use in children or for seizures. Still, Charlotte's situation was dire and Shackelford knew that she would die without any intervention, so he once again began poring over the research papers. One paper from 1980, by Raphael Mechoulam, caught his eye. In the paper, Mechoulam discusses "the effectiveness of giving synthesized cannabidiol or CBD to patients with seizures—in fact it was this particular molecule found in cannabis that shows therapeutic effects, without getting people high. In this paper 4 out of 8 people that used CBD became seizure free."[25] With this small but important bit of data Shackelford went about helping the Figis find a high–CBD oil to treat Charlotte. As we now know, the treatment was effective and Charlotte's story went on to kick off a huge influx of pediatric epilepsy patients to Colorado in search of CBD-oil treatment.

Even as Shackelford continued to treat his patients in Denver, he became more and more frustrated with the difficulties of studying cannabis in the U.S. Eventually the doctor decided to try to do research in Israel. In 2013 he visited the country and was able to speak with both Dr. Mechoulam and Dr. Yehuda Baruch, who at that time was the director of the Israeli Ministry of Health's Medical Cannabis Program.[26] After learning about the many studies occurring in Israel, Shackelford was further frustrated by the roadblocks to research back in the U.S. He was especially frustrated by the National Institute on Drug Abuse (NIDA)—one of the organizations that has to sign off on marijuana research—because it was "not interested in getting involved in medical marijuana research." In 2010 Shirley Simson, a spokesperson for the institute, told the *New York Times* the following: "As the National Institute on Drug Abuse, our focus is primarily on the negative consequences of marijuana use. We generally do not fund research focused on the potential beneficial medical effects of marijuana."[27] In 2014 (and up to the present day) that stance had not changed. Shackelford told an Israeli news site, "I knew I had to go somewhere else. I was very encouraged by my trip to Israel in early 2013 and decided I would come back."[28]

Dr. Shackelford has since completed the process for immigrating to Israel, although his commitments to his patients in Colorado mean that he splits his time between the two countries. He has cofounded a company called OWC (One World Cannabis) Pharmaceutical Research Corporation with Dr. Yehuda Baruch and is the chief science officer. As such, he has been granted permission to head up studies on "the efficacy of cannabis for patients with severe pain, seizures, cancer, migraines and PTSD."[29] In addition to allowing him to escape what he calls "the red tape" surrounding medical cannabis research in the United States,

Israel also offers Shackelford something that is nearly impossible to get in this country—a consistent product.

Until 2016 medical marijuana researchers in the U.S. had to use marijuana grown at the NIDA's facility at the University of Mississippi. The U.S. government formed the University of Mississippi's Marijuana Grow Project (M-Project) in 1968 to grow marijuana for research by the National Institute on Drug Abuse. The first plants were grown from Mexican seeds seized by the DEA. Since that time, all marijuana used in a federally approved study must come from the Mississippi site.[30] Although the DEA lifted its monopoly in 2016 no other institutions are yet federally licensed, so researchers must still use the Mississippi marijuana. The limited strains grown by the facility are provided to researchers as plant matter, meaning that oils and other products are not available. Also, marijuana is available only "in predetermined ratios of THC and CBD. None of the other cannabinoids—and there are at least 113 exhibiting varied effects—are available for research purposes."[31] Additionally, the quality of the marijuana available has come under question by researchers. In 2017, after waiting two years to get the cannabis she had requested for her approved PTSD study, Dr. Sue Sisley was shocked by what she received. She reported to PBS that when she opened the package to weigh the cannabis as required by the DEA it didn't resemble marijuana. "Most of it looked like green talcum powder."[32] Additionally, testing at independent laboratories in Colorado revealed the presence of mold in the plant material, and some samples did not match the chemical potency requested by the research team. "One sample, billed as having a 13 percent level of THC—the main psychoactive compound in marijuana—had just 8 percent when tested at the independent facility in Colorado. Other samples were off by lesser amounts."[33] Such discrepancies are a huge issue for researchers.

Meanwhile, Israel's more developed and regulated medical marijuana industry has been able to develop consistent products for research and use. This also means that the country is able to meet pharmaceutical standards and begin to create pharmaceutical-grade product from marijuana. Because there is no legal recreational market in Israel, all government-regulated marijuana grows are aimed for the medical market and growers work closely with doctors and scientists. Unlike in the United States (and Colorado), where doctors have little to no input into marijuana grows, in Israel "licensed marijuana growers work with scientific institutions in clinical trials toward the development of cannabis strains that treat a variety of illnesses and disorders."[34] This integrated, federally approved system leads to more and better research. There are currently 1,200 studies of medical cannabis occurring in Israel, looking at everything from autism to psoriasis.[35] Furthermore, regulated grows that work with scientists, in contrast to the fragmented system that exists in the United States, allow the investment necessary to develop pharmaceutical-grade product. The *Jerusalem Post* reported the following: "Israel boasts by far the most progressive regulatory environment for medical cannabis use worldwide. Most recently Israel's Health Ministry decided to allow distribution through pharmacies, driving the alignment of medical marijuana with other prescription drugs."[36] Meanwhile, federal regulations in the U.S. block rather than encourage research and development of cannabis medicine.

Such roadblocks have been a big problem for Dr. Nick Foreman, a pediatric oncologist from Children's Hospital in Denver who received one of nine grants from the Colorado Department of Health (CDPHE) for marijuana research. Because it is almost impossible to get federal grants to research the medical benefits of marijuana, in 2015 the board of health of the CDPHE made $9 million in grants available for marijuana research. The Medical Marijuana Scientific Advisory Council then recommended grants for nine studies, and the board approved the grants. While the majority of the grants went to Colorado researchers, there were also several out-of-state studies funded. Dr. Foreman received a little more than $1 million to study medical marijuana as palliative care in the pediatric brain tumor population. However, as mentioned above, while the grant money is certainly welcome in helping to find out more about cannabis and children's cancer care, federal regulations have presented multiple roadblocks to Dr. Foreman and his team.

As an oncologist, Dr. Foreman first became interested in marijuana for symptom relief in his clinical practice. Treating children with brain tumors is tough. Only about one-third of kids will survive, and, as many people know, the treatment is painful and difficult. In his gentle British accent, Dr. Foreman says, "We would do anything to reduce the side effects of our treatments on children." And for those children with untreatable forms of cancer, hospice care aims to make them as comfortable as possible in their remaining time. Even before legalization it was clear that cannabis provided good symptom relief for patients undergoing cancer treatment (particularly chemotherapy). However, Foreman had many questions: "Why do some children benefit but not others?" "Is it related to the child? Or the product?" "Is what people are saying about the product true?" and "What else is it doing (for example: affecting immune function?)." Additionally, although Marinol (synthetic THC) has long been available to treat cancer patients, it has never really shown much efficacy. Dr. Foreman gives the example of an ex-patient of his. The teenage boy was a 280-pound linebacker on his high school football team before starting cancer treatment for medulloblastoma, the most common malignant brain tumor in children. However, nausea and vomiting from his treatment caused him to drop to 135 pounds, and Marinol "was completely ineffectual." The boy went out on his own and got some marijuana, which he smoked in a joint. His nausea subsided, and with continued use of whole-plant cannabis he was able to get back up to 200 pounds.

With Marinol mostly ineffective and cannabis clearly having positive effects for some children, Dr. Foreman designed a multifaceted study to try to understand a bit more about cannabis and symptom control. However, this large, complex study almost immediately ran into problems due to the federal scheduling of the drug. One of the main issues is the fact that doctors cannot administer or prescribe marijuana as medicine. In fact, they can't even have the medicine in the hospital at all, so they cannot analyze what the patients are taking. Although they do test the metabolites in the patients' blood, they are otherwise reliant on parents' reporting of what they are giving their children. As Dr. Foreman points out, most of the time the parents don't know what is in the product because minimal regulation means lack of consistency. At one point, the researchers went out and toured some of the dispensaries providing product to their patients and found that the "claims of what is in the product are based in thin air." Not only does federal scheduling mean that the doctors must do observational rather than clinical studies (because they can't provide the drug), but also "not knowing what is in the product makes the studies much more limited."

Nick Foreman is not the only cannabis researcher in Colorado frustrated by research limitations. Dr. Kelly Knupp is a pediatric neurologist at Children's Hospital with a specialization in epilepsy. She generally sees the 30 percent of children whose epilepsy is not treatable through conventional means (those with disorders such as Dravet's syndrome). Because epilepsy was the first pediatric condition treated with cannabis in Colorado, Dr. Knupp has been fielding questions about marijuana from parents of patients for quite some time. In fact, after Charlotte's Web was featured on CNN, Knupp saw a "huge explosion" in interest and in people moving to the state. She says "the anecdotal reports of amazing responses were intriguing to everyone," and she completely understands why parents began to relocate to Colorado in attempts to cure their children. She says, "What parent wouldn't go to the moon and back for their child, and Colorado is not as far as the moon."

However, Dr. Knupp didn't really know what to tell parents about cannabis when they asked her, and she saw little evidence of its effectiveness outside of anecdotal reports. So, since she couldn't find the research, she decided to start undertaking it herself. The first thing her team did was a retrospective study—looking at how their patients who were using the drug were already doing. In the retrospective, which was later published, they found 30 percent to 50 percent of patients reporting some improvement in seizures, with no one actually seizure free.[37] There was a "disconnect" between their results and the anecdotes they were hearing from families. Dr. Knupp also saw an interesting trend: children who came to Colorado from outside the state to seek treatment were much more likely to report improvement than kids who already lived in Colorado. The research team wasn't able to account for this phenomenon but theorized that it could be a placebo effect or simply that a select group of patients were moving to the state. A second retrospective study showed results similar to the first.[38]

At this point, Dr. Knupp decided that they needed a prospective study that could compare patients before and after cannabis, as well as a control group not taking cannabis. She applied for and received a CDPHE grant to study cannabis and pediatric epilepsy. Like Dr. Foreman, she faced issues with her research right from the start. She says that she would have liked to have done a randomized, double-blind, placebo controlled study, "but you can't do that with an artisanal marijuana product." Once again, availability and quality of cannabis product was an issue for a medical marijuana study. NIDA provides its DEA-approved marijuana (from the University of Mississippi site) in plant form only for smoking (and it has been approved once for using with a vaporizer). However, almost every child who uses cannabis for medical purposes uses cannabis oil (some may take other edible forms), which essentially rules out a federally approved clinical study for children. As a Children's Hospital researcher, Dr. Knupp, like Dr. Foreman, cannot provide cannabis for her patients, test their cannabis product, or even allow them to bring it into the hospital. Thus, she depends on her patients to get their own medicine and report back to her. During her study, one of the constants that she hears from families is that the consistency of the cannabis products they buy varies each month, even for the exact same product. Knupp notes, "We really need a consistent product. The artisanal products that we have in Colorado are not pharmaceutical grade products."

While some researchers have a long wish list of changes they would like to see around marijuana policy and research, product regulation is at the very top of Kelly Knupp's list. She desperately wants to see Colorado's industry be more firmly regulated to produce a consistent medical product. She is concerned about the safety of her patients, saying that "families should know what they are getting and it should stay the same from month to month." She would also like to see state regulations that require distributors to follow up on patients and keep strict accounting of concentrations. Although, like many other researchers, she says the "FDA could make the process easier for people who are trying to do legitimate research," she also believes that the first step toward better research is a "consistent product."

Of course, inconsistency of product is only one problem faced by American researchers, even in legal states like Colorado. If doctors want to do a clinical trial rather than an observational study they must spend years going through a complex and convoluted process. Dr. Sue Sisley, a psychiatrist and former clinical assistant professor at the University of Arizona College of Medicine, had to wait seven years for approval to run a clinical study on cannabis and veterans with PTSD. Because marijuana is a Schedule I controlled substance with a long history of recreational use, the permitting process for medical research is much more difficult than for new pharmaceuticals.

The procedure for obtaining approval for a clinical study of cannabis involves seven steps. First the investigator must obtain a "pre-IND number from the FDA" ("IND" stands for "Investigational New Drug"—somewhat ironic in the case of cannabis, a drug that has been around for thousands of years). Then the research sponsor has to contact NIDA or another DEA-sponsored source "to obtain information on the specific strains of marijuana available, so that all necessary chemistry, manufacturing, and controls (CMC) information can be included in the IND application." As previously noted, the University of Mississippi is currently the only DEA-approved supplier. The research team must then contact the DEA for a registration application and a Schedule I license. Most of the time, the research sponsor then needs to obtain a letter of authorization (LOA) from NIDA to reference chemistry, manufacturing, and controls (CMC) information in NIDA's Drug Master File (DMF) on file with the DEA. Finally, researchers send a copy of the IND application and protocol (including the LOA) to the FDA and the DEA. The FDA then reviews the application and approves or denies the study. If the study passes through NIDA and the FDA, the DEA must then approve investigator registration and site licensure for the researchers and study sites. Research sponsors must next contact "NIDA or another DEA-registered source to obtain the marijuana after the FDA completes its review of the IND, and the DEA registration is received."[39] As if this process weren't complex enough, as previously noted NIDA is not generally interested in supporting research on the medical benefits of cannabis, preferring to focus on abuse and the negative side effects of the drug.

While studies on new pharmaceutical drugs must also pass through approval processes, the protocol is downright simple in comparison to the bureaucratic red tape faced by cannabis researchers. Essentially, drug developers must submit an IND application that includes information on the composition of the drug and the results of animal studies. The drug is then reviewed for approval for phase 1–3 trials in humans. Instead of erecting roadblocks to research, the FDA actually makes it as easy as possible to research new pharmaceuticals. Their website states, "Drug developers are free to ask for help from FDA at any point in the drug development process" and "FDA offers extensive technical assistance … [and] allows wide latitude in clinical trial design." Additionally, the FDA states that it will respond to IND submissions in 30 days with an approval or clinical hold and that "a clinical hold is rare."[40] An approval, of course, is just an approval for a clinical trial and does not mean that the drug will hit the market. Nevertheless, the far more complex process to research cannabis shows an inequity in the way in which the federal government approaches cannabis and pharmaceuticals.

Researchers and physicians have become increasingly frustrated over the years with the difficulty in doing clinical trials on cannabis, particularly as more and more states legalize medical marijuana and the products hit the market with little to no R&D. In 2016 scientists pressured the DEA to consider rescheduling cannabis as Schedule II or III to make research a bit easier. Sachin Patel, "an associate professor of psychiatry at Vanderbilt University School of Medicine who studies 'the role of endogenous cannabinoids as mediators of stress resiliency,' wanted to see cannabis moved to schedule II—drugs that are deemed to have medical use, but a high potential for abuse, like oxycodone or Percocet."[41] Dr. Patel told *Scientific American*, "Rescheduling cannabis as Schedule II will allow the research to get done that needs to be done to determine if this is going to be a good medicine, and for what."[42] Other scientists are in favor of less modest change. Dr. Chuanhai Cao, a cannabis researcher at the University of South Florida's Byrd Alzheimer's Institute, called for rescheduling to III, the group that includes drugs like Vicodin and Tylenol with codeine and that requires a much less arduous DEA approval process.[43] However, in August of 2016 the DEA announced that it would keep marijuana illegal for any purpose, retaining its Schedule I status.[44]

Despite the fact that the DEA has decided to maintain marijuana's status as a Schedule I drug, "with no currently accepted medical use and a high potential for abuse,"[45] a report from the National Academies of Sciences, Engineering, and Medicine released in early 2017 reaffirmed many medical uses of cannabis. The report "offers a rigorous review of scientific research published since 1999 about what is known about the health impacts of cannabis and cannabis-derived products." The 16 experts on the committee that published the report, including professors from top American medical colleges, considered more that 10,000 abstracts to reach their 100 conclusions. The committee had been tasked with examining the research on medical benefits of cannabis and the

U.S Drug Classification

SCHEDULE	DESCRIPTION	EXAMPLES
Schedule 1	Drugs with no currently accepted medical use and a high potential for abuse. These are the most dangerous drugs and may cause potentially severe psychological or physical dependence.	*Heroin *LSD *MDMA (Ecstasy) *Marijuana (cannabis)
Schedule 2	Drugs with a high potential for abuse, but some medical uses. These drugs are also considered dangerous.	*Cocaine *Methamphetamine *Methadone *Most opiates, including Vicodin, Dilaudid, Oxycontin *Dexedrine
Schedule 3	Drugs with a moderate to low potential for physical or psychological dependence.	*Ketamine *Tylenol with codeine *Anabolic steroids *Testosterone
Schedule 4	Drugs with a low potential for abuse and low risk of dependence.	*Xanax *Valium *Ativan *Ambien *Tramadol
Schedule 5	Drugs with the lowest potential for abuse. These drugs are generally used for antidiarrheal, antitussive or analgesic purposes.	*Cough medicines like Robitussin AC *Lomotil *Motofen *Lyrica

The United States Drug Scheduling System, with example drugs (Drug Enforcement Administration).

risks of use and abuse and to come up with "recommendations to help advance the research field and better inform public health decisions."[46]

In their conclusions the committee members came up with four recommendations to "support and improve the cannabis research agenda." First, the committee recommended addressing research gaps by developing a comprehensive national research agenda to "maximize the population-health impact of cannabis research." Secondly, they advised the improvement of research quality through "the development of guidelines for data collection, standards for research design and reporting, standardized terminology, and a minimum dataset for clinical and epidemiological studies." The third recommendation was to improve data collection through improved surveillance capacity. Fourth, and perhaps most important, the committee believed that research barriers must be addressed. As the report states, "The designation of cannabis as a Schedule I substance imposes numerous regulatory barriers that limit access to the funding and material resources necessary to conduct cannabis research." Among the suggestions toward righting the situation, the experts recommended the creation of a governmental committee made up of scientific experts, to be funded by "the Centers for Disease Control and Prevention, National Institutes of Health, U.S. Food and Drug Administration [FDA], industry groups, and nongovernmental organizations." The committee was tasked with the following:

• Proposing strategies for expanding access to research-grade marijuana, through the creation and approval of new facilities for growing and storing cannabis
• Identifying nontraditional funding sources and mechanisms to support a comprehensive national cannabis research agenda
• Investigating strategies for improving the quality, diversity, and external validity of research-grade cannabis products[47]

Clearly, this comprehensive report outlines the need for change in governmental policy in order to facilitate research. As long as marijuana remains a Schedule I drug, barriers to research will be difficult to overcome.

Even in Colorado, with its well-established medical marijuana industry and a medical system that is more accepting of cannabis as medicine, cannabis physicians and researchers continue to face obstacles. Like his fellow physicians at Children's Hospital in Denver, Dr. Nick Foreman and Dr. Kelly Knupp, Dr. Ed Hoffenberg received a grant from CPDHE to research cannabis and is encountering many of the same issues they are. Dr. Hoffenberg is a specialist in pediatric gastroenterology and director of the Center for Pediatric Inflammatory Bowel Diseases at Children's Hospital Colorado. He became interested in cannabis research when patients and their families began to ask him about the use of marijuana for IBDs such as Crohn's or told him they were already using the substance. So he applied for and received a grant to study the benefits of marijuana for juvenile patients with inflammatory bowel diseases. For the study, his team is following 105 enrolled patients from ages 13 to 23 and comparing those who use cannabis and those who don't use cannabis for disease characteristics—symptoms, quality of life, immune pathways, and potential mechanisms by which the use of marijuana might be helpful. They are also capturing data on motivations for use and potential side effects.

Like almost all of the other Colorado grant-funded cannabis studies, Dr. Hoffenberg's study is observational rather than clinical and faces many of the same issues involving drug inconsistency and Schedule I limitations. In fact, Hoffenberg and his team wrote an article, published in the *Journal of Pediatric Gastroenterology and Nutrition*, outlining the state of medical marijuana in Colorado and his study on cannabis and IBD and highlighting "the challenges federal laws impose on conducting research on cannabis and IBD." The article states that while Colorado's legalization has opened up some new possibilities for medical research, "academic researchers in Colorado now face some paradoxical challenges because under federal law, cannabis continues to remain a Schedule 1 drug."[48] The authors then go on to list a variety of challenges, including uncertainty about the future of legal cannabis in Colorado due to changes at the federal level, continued risk of being involved in litigation, and lack of funding sources. Also, the article discusses that at "universities receiving Title IV federal student aid funding, the Drug-Free Schools and Campuses Regulations (EDGAR Part 86) require the implementation of a program to prevent the unlawful possession, use, or distribution of illicit drugs and alcohol by students and employees, and a policy that stipulates that a student or employee who violates the alcohol and other drugs policy is subject to both the institution's sanction and to criminal sanction provided by federal, state, and local law."[49] Since Children's Hospital is affiliated with the University of Colorado, this regulation imposes further challenges to research. The university, in trying to avoid conflict with federal law, compiled a long list of "guidelines" for cannabis research in February of 2016, further limiting research faculty (see Appendix A for the full guidelines).

Hoffenberg et al.'s article goes on to discuss issues with obtaining and using consistent cannabis products for research. The authors note that despite the fact that "many observational studies would benefit from having a quantitative analysis of the various CBs in the product(s) used by the end users," FDA and DEA regulations mean "researchers are not allowed to have patients bring their cannabis products on campus for chemical analysis, and the state-certified laboratories only perform testing for licensed cannabis growers."[50] Like other Colorado researchers I spoke with, Dr. Hoffenberg reiterated in an interview that one of the major limitations with his study is that the researchers really don't know what the patients are actually taking. They can't test the product or "manipulate the subjects' use of marijuana," so they are completely dependent on blood tests of metabolites and the patients' (and their families') self-reporting. In Dr. Hoffenberg's case, these limitations are extremely crucial because after examining the cannabis research that has been done on this topic he found very limited data. There have been only "3 observational studies of approximately 300 adult subjects," and "a single placebo-controlled clinical trial of THC was conducted for treatment of Crohn's disease." All of these showed promising results. However, there are no studies examining the effects of cannabis on children with IBD. Clearly, Hoffenberg's research is vital and could benefit from fewer limitations.

While opponents of medical marijuana often cite a lack of research as a reason for continued prohibition, it seems that cannabis researchers are caught between a rock and a hard place. As the National Academies of Sciences report shows, there has been a substantial amount of research already done on marijuana; but it is true that quality double-blind, placebo-controlled trials are lacking. Yet the Schedule I status of marijuana still hampers clinical research due to massive red tape, lack of funding, and an inadequate supply of consistent cannabis medicine. Even in legal states like Colorado physicians continue to struggle against research roadblocks. While Dr. Nick Foreman hopes that his study on medical marijuana and cancer in children can help to add to the fairly small body of knowledge about pediatric cannabis care, he is frustrated by its limitations. He says that the "scheduling is completely mad" and "all of this research should have been done 20–30 years ago." He, like all of the researchers I spoke with, would also like to see a more regulated marijuana industry in Colorado and other states so that patients truly know what product they are taking. In the meantime, while opponents argue against medical marijuana on the basis of a lack of research, physicians like Foreman continue to struggle against the system in order to do that research, and hopefully, alleviate some of the pain and suffering of their patients.

CHAPTER 6

Thank You for Your Service

On December 24, 2009, Matt Kahl decided he didn't want to live anymore. He took every drug in the house, whether prescribed or over-the-counter: Advil, Aleve, mood stabilizers, Percocet and more. Then he lay down on the couch to die. When his wife found him, he was no longer breathing. She called an ambulance, and the EMTs were able to revive him and stabilize his vitals. He was then medevacked to Vanderbilt Hospital in Nashville, the closest major hospital to Ft. Campbell, Kentucky, where Matt was stationed at the time with the storied 101st Airborne unit. Fortunately, Matt recovered quickly, and he was soon back at work on the base. Because the suicide attempt had happened over Christmas break, the rest of his unit didn't realize he had tried to take his life and he brushed the overdose off, telling them, "I'm fine. It was an accident." In such a prestigious unit, suicide, or mental illness in general, is perceived as an unmanly weakness, so Matt continued to put up a "strong front." Just eight months after that first suicide attempt, he was deployed for the second time to Afghanistan.

Matt's journey into the desperation that led him to try to kill himself started many years before. His father was a colonel in the Marines, and Matt spent his childhood moving from base to base around the world—Japan, Norway, Germany, and the U.S. Eventually he ended up in North Carolina, where he went to high school and later attended Appalachian State University, and studied behavioral neuroscience. After graduating, he stayed in North Carolina working in various fields, including audio engineering. Because of a somewhat conflicted relationship with his father, Matt never thought he would join the military. However, after 9/11, the start of the war in the Middle East, and the birth of his son, he felt compelled to "defend the principles of the United

States; put simply, freedom, individual freedom." Because he was older by this point, age 29, he no longer qualified for the Marines and instead went to the Raleigh Military Entrance Processing Station (MEPS) and enlisted in the army. More than anything, he wanted to be on the front lines, to "fight a war."

Thus, when Matt scored the maximum score on the ASVAB (the military aptitude test), he turned down a variety of the jobs offered to him. He wanted to fight, not repair vehicles or make deliveries. So when he was offered a position in infantry he took it. He was shipped out to basic training at Ft. Benning Infantry School, after which he and his family were stationed at Ft. Campbell and he was assigned to the 101st Airborne Division. He thought he might become an officer one day, but he wanted to start out on the front lines—to be where the action was. And he soon would be. He left for his first deployment in 2008. Once he got to Afghanistan life was tough, but Matt did well; he was older and more educated than most soldiers in his unit, and he became the "go to guy" for a little while. But he incurred a multitude of undiagnosed head injuries during that first deployment. Matt recalls one occasion when he was lying behind a berm with his ear pressed to the ground to try to stay as flat as possible. A rocket-propelled grenade (RPG) hit the ground on the other side of the berm, and he ended up losing most of his hearing in that ear. Additionally, he suffered from migraines and vomiting for days afterwards. Multiple veterans have told me that the military wasn't really tracking traumatic brain injuries (TBIs) in Afghanistan or Iraq, so soldiers usually just got a day of bed rest and were then sent back out on patrol. Matt recalls that he probably had six or seven concussions (mild TBIs) during his first deployment.

Medical science has now demonstrated the unfortunate possible long-term negative health effects of concussions, particularly repeated TBIs. While most people know that vomiting, dizziness, and headaches are all immediate signs of concussion, many other symptoms may not appear for days, weeks, or even months. After suffering a TBI, a person may experience visual disturbances, memory loss, poor attention and concentration, sleep disturbances, vertigo, loss of balance, irritability and emotional disturbances, feelings of depression, mood changes, slowness in thinking, or even seizures.[1] These symptoms are even more likely to appear if the patient suffers repeated TBIs, and cumulative concussions are "known to cause increased risk for prolonged or permanent neurologic damage, including early onset dementia."[2] Additionally, the true effects of TBIs on the veterans of the last 20 years are only now starting to be seen. Traumatic brain injury has been called the "signature wound" of the Iraq and Afghanistan wars. One study showed "nearly a third of all combat injuries treated at the Walter Reed Army Medical Center (WRAMC) in early 2008 involved TBI and that ~20 percent of patients evacuated by air from the Operation Iraqi Freedom (OIF) combat zone were classified as having at least a head or neck injury."[3] And these estimates are probably low, as every veteran I spoke with mentioned that head injury was extremely common among their fellow soldiers.

When Matt Kahl returned from Afghanistan in 2009 he felt that his first deployment had gone "extremely well." He says he felt fine for the first few months or so, but the brain injuries had done their damage. His health soon began to deteriorate, and he sought relief from his physical and mental injuries in the prescriptions the army gave him, including opiate narcotics and psychoactive medications. He also began to seek relief in alcohol. He withdrew from his wife and was angry and irritable, lashing out at his family. He couldn't tell them what was wrong because, as he now says, "I didn't know myself." His anguish reached a peak that holiday season, and he made his first suicide attempt. Unfortunately, he did not receive psychological help after his overdose, as he insisted to his family and the military that he was fine. However, he "really didn't have a will to live," so in August of 2010 he signed up to go back to Afghanistan and was soon volunteering for the most dangerous assignments.

On his second deployment it didn't take long for Matt to be injured again. His unit received the news that one of their medics had been shot and killed while shielding a downed soldier. Matt set out with a group of his colleagues to bring back the medic's body and retrieve the rest of the soldiers. Although his memory from those years is jumbled, a common symptom of both TBIs and PTSD, he does remember that they were rolling out at high speed for the rescue mission when there was a "loud boom." Matt was a gunner in the turret, so when the explosion happened he flew forward and smashed into the turret shield, a half-inch steel plate. The vehicle was traveling about 30 miles an hour, and his face and jaw were smashed before he flew through the air and landed on his head, instantaneously losing consciousness. He was medevacked from that operation to receive treatment for his multiple injuries, including damage to his face, a fracture in his jaw, ruptured discs in his cervical spine, and damage to his lumbar-sacral spine. Also, he was finally diagnosed with a traumatic brain injury. The mental issues he had been suffering from before worsened in the hospital, where he was dealing with almost constant anxiety attacks. The doctors noticed, and they finally began to talk with him seriously about PTSD.

Post-traumatic stress disorder was first recognized in 1980, when it was added to the American Psychiatric Association's *Diagnostic and Statistical Manual of Mental Disorders*. The National Institutes of Health defines PTSD as an "anxiety disorder that some people develop after seeing or living through an event that caused or threatened serious harm or death." It is estimated to affect approximately 7.7 million adults per year in the U.S., although the disorder can also develop in children.[4] Those with PTSD may suffer a wide variety of symptoms, although the syndrome is characterized by reliving the event in nightmares or flashbacks (also called reexperiencing symptoms). PTSD sufferers often experience anxiety in situations similar to the one that triggered the disorder and may avoid situations or people that trigger memories of the event. Additional symptoms of PTSD include depression, insomnia, trouble concentrating, moodiness and irritability, and even angry outbursts and rage. While only subtle symptoms may show up immediately after the triggering event, more severe symptoms can emerge many months later. Current treatments include psychotherapy and selective serotonin reuptake inhibitors (SSRIs) such as Paxil and Zoloft.[5] However, many people with PTSD, especially in more severe forms, do not find relief from these conventional treatments.

In addition to a lack of suitable treatments, PTSD sufferers also have to deal with the stigma associated with the condition. Post-traumatic stress disorder was "once considered a psychological condition of combat veterans who were 'shocked' by and unable to face their experiences on the battlefield."[6] There was much debate among the public about whether it was in fact a "real" disorder, and soldiers who suffered from it often were rejected by their peers and seen as weak. Today, even with much greater knowledge about the condition, many of these stigmas live on. It is still considered largely a soldiers' condition (with approximately 20 percent of combat soldiers and veterans diagnosed with it), but we now know that it affects not only survivors of "combat experience, but also terrorist attacks, natural disasters, serious accidents, assault or abuse, or even sudden and major emotional losses."[7] Nonetheless, PTSD remains associated primarily with military veterans, and much of the shame associated with "weakness" and "mental illness" persists in these settings. In my interviews with veterans, they all talked about not wanting to admit that they could have PTSD or somehow feeling that they could just work their way through it. There was a sense that they would "let down their unit" if they were diagnosed with PTSD or that their peers would no longer see them as "tough."

Matt Kahl is no exception to this rule, which is why it took him two deployments and multiple traumatic events before he would even talk seriously with a doctor about PTSD. By the time he was diagnosed with the disorder he had already experienced symptoms of anxiety and depression for months if not years. Yet, although the doctor convinced him he needed to focus on himself for his own sake and the sake of his family, he still rued the diagnosis. Afterwards, he recalls, his unit "treated me like crap," and he began to sink down into a deep, dark hole. Even though he was now receiving treatment for the PTSD it wasn't working, and his symptoms worsened. He suffered from feelings of hopelessness and abandonment. He was anxious and consistently worried that "someone would shoot a bullet through the wall of my house." Matt became more and more despondent, until, in 2011, he tried to kill himself for the second time. Once more he survived, but this time the military took note and he was given a general discharge under honorable conditions.

At the end of that year, feeling "abandoned, broken and used up," Matt moved to North Carolina to be with his wife, who was having their second child. By this point his doctors had him on what he now calls "an ungodly amount of drugs," 18 to 20 prescription medications a month. Today he can't even remember all of the medications, but he does remember being on several pain meds, 2 benzodiazepines, 3–4 neuroleptics, one SSRI and various other drugs to counter the side effects from these primary medications. He was also being prescribed off-label drugs for his PTSD, including an antipsychotic medication called Seroquel, which is generally prescribed for mental diseases such as psychosis, bipolar disorder, and schizophrenia—none of which Matt Kahl suffered. Looking back, he is astounded by the number and types of drugs the military (and later the VA) doctors prescribed for him. For example, despite his two suicide attempts, doctors prescribed him both Zoloft and Paxil, SSRIs that studies have shown "may cause worsening of suicidal ideas in vulnerable patients."[8]

By the time Matt moved back to North Carolina, he recalls, he was "detached, unable to make any kind of connection with anyone around me." When his son was born he says he felt nothing; he didn't even want to hold the baby. Like so many patients who end up trying

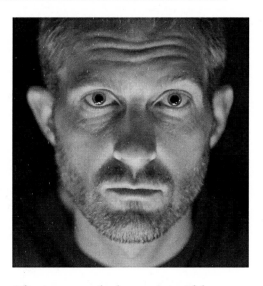

After two army deployments to Afghanistan, where he suffered traumatic brain injury (TBI), Matt Kahl suffered from severe PTSD that made him suicidal. He later moved to Colorado, where treatment with cannabis controlled his disorder (courtesy Charles Shaw, from *Soldiers of the Vine,* 2017, Charles Shaw, director).

cannabis, Matt's massive quantity of powerful prescriptions had turned him into a zombie. Additionally, they weren't really helping much with his pain, neurodegenerative disorder, or PTSD. Fortunately, around this time he started getting treatment from doctors at Camp Lejeune Marine Base, where he recalls receiving very good care. He saw a doctor with the Defense Veterans Brain Injury Center (DVBIC) for his TBIs and decided to ask him about marijuana, which Matt had heard could help with pain and PTSD. To his surprise, the doctor said, "Well, you can try it, and if you don't like it, just don't do it." So Matt bought some marijuana on the black market and tried it. While many of his memories from that time period are hazy, he can remember that first time smoking a joint very clearly. He says that it worked almost immediately to alleviate his PTSD and anxiety. He remembers a "blissful" feeling coming over him as the tenseness he constantly carried just melted away.

At this point Matt decided he needed to move to a state where medical marijuana was legal in order to access what was clearly the most effective treatment he had tried. His wife saw how much the cannabis helped him, so she agreed as well. In June 2013 they packed up their belongings and moved with their two sons to Colorado. Matt was able to get a medical card within a week due to his record of chronic pain (since PTSD was still not a qualifying condition at the time). He remembers the first time he went to meet with his VA doctor in Colorado. He decided to ask him about marijuana, knowing that even though it was legal in the state it was still not federally legal or approved by the VA. Again, a doctor surprised him: "If you haven't tried it, you probably should, but I can't give you these other drugs while you are on medical marijuana." Matt didn't hesitate to reply: "Fine. Take me off of these opiate narcotics."

As with most patients who have been on high amounts of narcotics, the withdrawals weren't easy but the marijuana certainly helped. To this day, Matt has no regrets about trading in his pharmaceuticals for cannabis. "It was the best thing I ever did. I never looked back." In North Carolina his pain and neurodegenerative disorder had been so bad that even with his multiple prescriptions he ended up in a wheelchair. However, after starting cannabis Matt was able to get out of the chair and start using a walker and then a cane. Finally, in April of 2015, he was able to give up the cane. Now he hardly even has a limp. Prior to using medical marijuana, Matt also had frequent neuralgia—shooting pains in his face due to the nerve damage there. These, too, have nearly disappeared since he started cannabis therapy. Due to his multiple TBIs, Matt once suffered from frequent and debilitating migraines; today his migraines have decreased from three to five times a week to one every few months. All in all, his pain and neurodegenerative disorder are greatly improved.

Perhaps one of Matt's biggest improvements since the start of marijuana treatment, however, has been mental. His PTSD is much more controlled with the use of cannabis. Nowadays he doesn't suffer from the debilitating depression and mood changes associated with the disorder. Additionally, he says that he no longer feels cut off from the world. He has been able to get off of all of his pharmaceuticals and is not using anything but cannabis for his various medical conditions. Cannabis also led him into the world of community building and activism. He started out by giving his extra marijuana to other veterans, but soon saw a need for community and education and joined in with the organization Weed for Warriors, an organization started by a Marine Corps veteran in the San Francisco Bay area to "provide Veterans with medical marijuana information, a safe place for fellowship with other Veterans and safe access to free medicine with proof of service/current medical recommendation."[9] He now runs his own organization, called Veterans for Natural Rights, whose mission is, in his words, "to change policy by creating a space where veterans can heal, find their voice, and change the world." Matt was also an outspoken advocate to add PTSD to the official list of medical conditions in Colorado. He feels that of all of his medical conditions, PTSD was the most debilitating and he "knew how much marijuana helped with it." Like many other refugees who make their way to Colorado and find healing with this plant, Matt is now dedicated to making sure healing is available for others.

Unfortunately, Matt Kahl is not alone in finding himself disabled physically and mentally after returning from war. Physical disability, TBIs, PTSD, depression, and suicide are endemic conditions among the veteran population. In 2013, ten years after the start of the war in Iraq and 12 years after the start of the war in Afghanistan, the numbers were already staggering. While over 6,600 Americans were killed in Afghanistan and Iraq, the numbers affected after returning home to the U.S. are much larger. Over 2.5 million members of the army, navy, air force, Marines, coast guard and reserve and national guard units served in these two wars, and over a third were deployed multiple times.[10] Although far more soldiers were killed in the Vietnam War, disability claims per veteran for Afghanistan and Iraq have already risen above any other U.S. war. Of the approximately 1.6 million military members from those wars who have transitioned to veteran status, 670,000 have been awarded disability status and over 100,000 have claims pending.[11]

Possibly the most disturbing statistic of all involves the number of veterans who commit suicide. Approximately 20 percent of all suicides in the U.S. are veterans, even though vets only make up about 9 percent of the population.[12] A Department of Veterans Affairs study completed in 2016 showed that the veteran suicide rate had risen sharply since 2001: totaling 35 percent for all veterans and an alarming 85 percent for female vets.[13] The study also showed that roughly 20 veterans commit suicide every day, with over 7,400 vets taking their own lives in 2014 alone.[14] While this number is a decrease from the 22 suicides a day cited by the VA in 2012, the reality is that suicide rates are not decreasing; there are just fewer veterans in all than there were at that time. Suicide rates overall are increasing in the United States, and the rate among veterans is over twice as high as the civilian rate. The *New York Times* reported as follows: "Hardest hit were young veterans. The suicide rate for veterans age 18 to 29 was 86 deaths per 100,000 for men and 33 deaths per 100,000 for women—much higher than previous estimates, and almost twice as high as all other age groups. The civilian suicide rate is about 14 deaths per 100,000."[15] Suicide rates are only the tip of the iceberg. The Department of Defense reports 361,092 traumatic brain injuries in the military from 2000 to 2016.[16] Since every veteran I spoke with told me that TBIs were common and underreported during active duty, the actual numbers are almost certainly higher. Along with TBI statistics, PTSD numbers, which are also most likely underreported due to the stigmas discussed earlier, are extremely high. The Department of Veterans Affairs estimates that between 15 and 20 percent of Gulf War veterans suffer from PTSD, while the percentage for Vietnam vets is closer to 30 percent.[17]

The numbers of veterans suffering from mental trauma are staggering, but the government is not ignoring the matter. In addition to the above studies, the VA has, in recent years, "hired 5,300 mental health providers and support personnel and upgraded its Veterans Crisis Line in response to the problem."[18] Additionally, the Defense and Veterans Brain Injury Center has existed since 1992 and has collaborated with the VA and various medical organizations for extensive research into brain injury and treatment. In recent years the military and VA have given more attention to TBIs and PTSD in an attempt to deal with the current crisis, but they are still behind the curve. Renowned veterans' benefits lawyer Katrina Eagle told me, "The VA is one of the world's leading researchers and providers for prosthetic limbs, but they are one of the last for researching and understanding injuries to the brain." Thus, many veterans who aren't finding the treatment they need through the VA are striking out on their own and networking with other vets to find effective treatments, including federally illegal cannabis.

One of those veterans is Rocky Hall. When the U.S. invaded Iraq on the evening of Rocky's 19th birthday, March 19, 2003, he took it as a sign that he should join the army. A Texas native, Rocky enlisted in 2004 and was sent to Fort Bragg in North Carolina. Hall recounts, "Where I'm from, you either go to work or you go to war; I chose war." After his training, his unit—3/321 FA 18th Airborne Corp—was sent to the Middle East. He was deployed to Iraq in 2005 and suffered his first traumatic brain injury after being thrown 25 feet when the Humvee he was riding in exploded. He was then sent back to North Carolina, where he immediately began treatment and TBI rehab. He was in and out of the hospital at UNC/Raleigh, seeing neurologists for severe symptoms that included acute vertigo. If he stood up to walk he would "just fall down," so he had to use a walker for about nine months. After one year of treatment at Ft. Bragg and UNC for his traumatic brain injury, Hall was reclassified into a noncombat Military Occupational Specialty (MOS) in the chemical, nuclear, biological field.

Unfortunately, being in a noncombat MOS didn't mean an end to Hall's injuries. After a 2009 deployment to Iraq he suffered another TBI while training with his unit at Ft. Hood, Texas. His vertigo returned, along with slurred speech. He was sent to the speech pathology and TBI clinic in Ft. Hood for further treatment. At around this same time, Rocky had the bad luck of being in the wrong place at the wrong time. On November 5, 2009, he was waiting to be seen at the Ft. Hood TBI clinic. At the same time, U.S. Army major and psychiatrist Nidal Hassan entered the attached Soldier Readiness Processing Center, where army personnel receive routine treatment before and after deployment. Hassan approached the front desk, bowed down, shouted "Allahu Akbar," and opened fire, killing 13 people and injuring more than 30 others.[19] Rocky Hall was not in the same room as the shooting, but he was in the same building. The traumatic event, combined with his multiple TBIs, would end up causing him to develop severe PTSD.

Hall's troubles did not end there. Later, as an airborne paratrooper, he did multiple jumps while stationed with the 3rd MISB (A) at Ft. Bragg, North Carolina, and the 10th SFG (A) at Ft. Carson, Colorado. He then developed a neuro-spasticity problem on the right side of his body due to his previous TBIs and traumatic injury of the parietal lobe of his brain. These injuries would eventually turn into a seizure disorder, causing him to be medically separated from military service. The army tried to treat Hall's multiple injuries and mental issues. Although he believes he did receive some good treatment, including being part of brain injury studies and innovative therapies through the Defense Brain Institute, his health continued to decline. He developed degenerative disk disease, which caused him almost constant pain. His PTSD produced a variety of mental symptoms including insomnia, anger, and depression. In addition, his moodiness and irritability contributed to divorce from his wife, whom he had met while training in 2007. They became engaged while they were both deployed in Iraq and were married in 2009, a month after the Hassan shooting. In attempts to deal with his many symptoms, doctors prescribed him dozens of pharmaceuticals, including synthetic opiate narcotics like Dilaudid, massive doses of Neurontin for pain, Klonopin (an antipsychotic benzodiazepine) and antidepressants. Not only did the prescriptions not provide relief, they actually made things worse. In fact, he developed multiple side effects including extreme nausea and diarrhea, causing him to no longer be able to eat and to lose massive amounts of weight. As he recalls, "I was wasting away." Finally, when his neurologist found out that he was being medically separated from the army, she recommended that he contact Sue Sisley and Veterans for Natural Rights about using cannabis for his condition. It was casual advice, but it would end up changing his life.

Rocky knew he wanted to explore marijuana for his medical conditions. He was even allowed to attend a "Veterans to Farmers" program in Denver as part of his transition into civilian life. He had heard that in Texas the VA stop benefits if they find marijuana in a vet's system, whereas in Colorado one only needed to find a doctor to agree with that treatment plan. Rocky's concern about losing benefits is a common one among vets who use, or are considering using, medical cannabis, but it does not seem to have a basis in real policy. In a letter sent on June 2, 2017, to Veterans Affairs director David Shulkin, Representative J. Luis Correa, a Democrat from California and member of the House Veterans Affairs Committee, claimed that veterans had told them they were being denied treatment at VA facilities if they tested positive for THC in their systems "in states where it is legal and they have a doctor's prescription."[20] The VA responded officially as follows: "Veterans will not be denied care for all appropriate conditions including medical, behavioral and substance abuse conditions. Veterans who are participating in state medical marijuana programs can continue getting the treatment based on the medically approved protocols as prescribed by the approved physicians in the respective states. Veterans can concurrently get care at the VA."[21] While it is unclear what the VA's policy has been about medical marijuana in legal states in the past, in a personal interview Katrina Eagle, a lawyer whose specialty is veterans' benefits, told me that in her 20 years of work with veterans she had neither seen nor heard of a veteran having benefits pulled for having a medical marijuana card. Additionally, the VA's 2017 statement claims that the organization will not interfere with a vet's marijuana treatment in the future.

In any case, Rocky Hall's doctors in Colorado recognized the terrible side effects of his pharmaceuticals and helped him wean himself off of the drugs. Meanwhile, he got his medical card and started to use medical-grade cannabis regularly. The results were overwhelmingly positive. The cannabis, which he smokes or drinks in lemonade form, helped to relieve the pain from his degenerative disk problem so that he could become more mobile again. Additionally, it helped with his pain and anxiety. Whereas previously he would find himself isolated in his house, unable to face the anxiety associated with big buildings in public places (he would often face anxiety after pulling up to his gym, for example), he now had energy and wanted to go out and be active. Before starting cannabis Hall would drink himself to sleep just to deal with the unrelenting pain and PTSD. Now he rarely drinks and he has managed to wean himself off of all the pharmaceuticals. In regard to his PTSD, Rocky says that the cannabis helped him to rethink his anxiety: "Like the Dewey Decimal system, I can re-organize my brain—shut the door that doesn't need to be open."

Rocky Hall and Matt Kahl are just two of the thousands of veterans who have been helped by medical marijuana. While cannabis shows promise for a variety of conditions that plague vets, from chronic pain to nerve issues, one of the most significant uses for the drug appears to be in combatting PTSD. As previously noted, there are few, if any, effective treatments for this debilitating mental condition. Still, opponents of medical marijuana note that little research has been done on marijuana and PTSD and reports of its efficacy are anecdotal. They fear that vets may be trading dependencies on pharmaceuticals for addiction to another drug. In fact, the VA's own PTSD website calls dependency on marijuana "cannabis use disorder" and lists among its symptoms psychosis, poor life satisfaction, and addiction with a "clinically significant withdrawal syndrome" (oddly, the Veterans Affairs website lacks consistency in its messages about marijuana. In fact, it often has completely contradictory statements about cannabis from one page to another). The reality, despite any claims on the VA's website, is that while there has not been much research on cannabis and PTSD in the past (due mostly to the drug's Schedule I status), the scientific community is beginning to look much more seriously at the plant for dealing with PTSD and associated conditions. Even the VA itself has begun to admit the possibilities of cannabis as treatment for veterans. In June of 2017 VA secretary David Shulkin addressed the organization's willingness to examine the medical value of marijuana in his "State of the VA" speech. While he noted that the VA could not prescribe medical marijuana while it is still illegal under federal law, he did say the following: "There may be some evidence that this is beginning to be helpful. And we're interested in looking at that and learning from that."[22]

Other organizations have also begun to hear veterans' calls for help, as more and more groups like Weed for Warriors and Veterans for Natural Rights have formed to advocate for legal medical cannabis. Even the usually conservative American Legion, the nation's largest veterans' organization, is pressuring the government to make cannabis more readily available for medical research. In May 2017 the Legion posted an article on Defense One, a defense community website, entitled "What Wounded Veterans Need: Medical Marijuana." The article's authors, Joe Plenzler and Lou Celli, note "many Afghanistan and Iraq veterans have contacted the American Legion to relay their personal stories about the efficacy of cannabis in significantly improving their quality of life by enabling sleep, decreasing the prevalence of night terrors, mitigating hyper-alertness, reducing chronic pain, and more." They also cite findings by the congressionally mandated National Academies of Sciences, Engineering, and Medicine that there is "conclusive or substantial evidence that cannabis or cannabinoids are effective for the treatment of chronic pain, reducing nausea and vomiting during chemotherapy, and lowering spasticity in multiple sclerosis sufferers, that there is 'moderate evidence'" that cannabis is effective in treating sleep apnea, fibromyalgia, and chronic pain, and "limited evidence" that cannabis improves symptoms of post-traumatic stress disorder and creates better outcomes after traumatic brain injury.[23] It is clear that the scientific, veteran, and even political communities are starting to recognize the potential of cannabis as medicine.

While the National Academies of Sciences, Engineering, and Medicine study's findings on PTSD are based on only one "small, fair-quality trial," more studies are on the way. In 2016 government agencies finally approved a PTSD and cannabis trial by principal investigator Dr. Sue Sisley, a psychiatrist and former clinical assistant professor at the University of Arizona College of Medicine. Dr. Sisley's research has primarily focused on medical uses of marijuana, and the new study is a "Placebo-Controlled, Triple-Blind, Randomized Crossover Pilot Study of the Safety and Efficacy of Four Different Potencies of Smoked Marijuana in 76 Veterans with Chronic, Treatment-Resistant Posttraumatic Stress Disorder."[24] Unfortunately, the road to approval for this PTSD study has been a long and rocky one. Dr. Sisley first began discussing the study with her colleague Rick Doblin way back in 2009. Through the Multidisciplinary Association for Psychedelic Studies (MAPS) they applied for an Investigational New Drug number for marijuana (THC and CBD) from the Food and Drug Administration (FDA). This was the only way to be allowed to legally conduct a clinical study of a drug on the Schedule I list. They received the number in November 2010, but one month later the study was put on hold because the FDA said they had not provided the "manufacturer" of the marijuana. This was only one of the many roadblocks that both the FDA and the National Institute on Drug Abuse would attempt to put in the way of the MAPS PTSD study.[25]

MAPS requested the marijuana to be used in the study from NIDA (the government's farmed marijuana in Mississippi) and was told in early 2011 that NIDA would provide them with the drug. Only one month later, however, the investigators received a letter from the FDA indicating seven issues related to protocol design of the study. One week later the researchers had a teleconference with the FDA to address these concerns, including the potential diversion of marijuana from the study to the public. MAPS submitted the revised protocol one month later and it was accepted by the FDA and sent on to the Department of Health and Human Services (HHS) to be reviewed by NIDA and the Public Health Service (PHS). In mid-2011, after a nearly five-month wait, HHS informed the researchers that the protocol had been unanimously rejected by the NIDA/PHS reviewers. While the issues the reviewers had with the protocol are too complex to enumerate here, suffice it to say that the researchers were not about to give up. The following year they got approval from the Institutional Review Board (IRB) at the University of Arizona, Dr. Sisley's employing university. With this new approval and various changes, they resubmitted the protocol to HHS in 2014 and it was approved.[26]

Unfortunately, this approval would not be the end in the struggle to conduct this clinical trial. Just one month later NIDA said that, despite its assurances in 2011, it did not have the marijuana for the study and would "need to grow a new crop." Then three months later, in the biggest blow to the research yet, Dr. Sue Sisley was fired from the University of Arizona. While the university denied that the firing was for political reasons or had anything to do with her cannabis research, Dr. Sisley does not agree. She told the Los Angeles Times "she was fired after her research—and her personal political crusading—created unwanted attention for the university from legislative Republicans who control its purse strings." Dr. Sisley continued her explanation: "This is a clear political retaliation for the advocacy and education I have been providing the public and lawmakers. I pulled all my evaluations and this is not about my job performance."[27] Sisley's termination was a huge setback to the study, since she had spent months persuading the research board at the university to approve it. She had to start the process anew.

Dr. Sisley and her co-investigators would spend the next two years getting IRB approval from the co-investigators' home universities (University of Pennsylvania and Johns Hopkins University) and from the new Arizona study location—a private clinic in Phoenix. Finally, in April 2016, the study received DEA approval for the Baltimore and Phoenix trial sites—the last step in the long government approval process. Of prime importance was the fact that before receiving final governmental approval the study received a grant in December 2014 (six months after Dr. Sisley was fired) from the Colorado Department of Public Health and Environment for the full cost of the study—$2.156 million.[28] Because it is so difficult to receive funding from the federal government for studies on Schedule I drugs, Colorado's grants for medical cannabis research were a key component in making this PTSD study possible and have shown the influence of Colorado's laws far beyond the state's borders.

Zach Phillips is one veteran who moved to Colorado in part because of Dr. Sisley's influence. Zach originally joined the navy in 2004 to "see the world, be challenged and have new experiences," and he had been deployed with amphibious operations. He traveled all over the world on deployments—the Middle East, the Mediterranean, the Persian Gulf, and other locations. On one deployment in the Red Sea he discovered a fire in the middle of the night. A trained first responder, Zach was rushing down a ladder when he fell down the ladder well, injuring his back on the bottom steps. He was supposed to go to a hospital in Bahrain, but the ship did not end up stopping there. He had to "tough out" the last three months of his deployment until they returned to the U.S. When he arrived at his home base in Virginia Beach, he was immediately sent to the Portsmouth Naval Hospital. It was 2007 and the doctors decided to pull him off the ship due to his injuries. His deployments were over.

When Zach tries to remember that time in his life, it is all "a blur." He remembers that he "had just gotten back from cheating death on three separate occasions on deployment" and his wife was having severe mental issues, acting like a "Jekyll and Hyde," as he puts it. Later they would find out she was dying of brain cancer (which had been misdiagnosed for three years). Meanwhile, he was also dealing with plenty of health problems of his own. His back injury would cause him temporary paralysis. He had to use a walker (and later a wheelchair) because his knees would just buckle and he would fall to the ground. Additionally, like many other vets, he soon found himself on "heavy pharmaceuticals, over half of which were narcotics." In an all-too-common story, Zach started drinking heavily to aid with the pain and to help him go to sleep at night. He says that the next thing he knew he was drinking "a 1.75 handle of rum or vodka every night to help him fall asleep, and then getting up every morning at 4:30 to be out at the base by six. Nothing fazed me." At this point Zach's doctor referred him to a psychiatrist who diagnosed him with insomnia and PTSD and added Valium and sleeping pills to his pharmaceutical cocktail.

After leaving the service, Zach decided to move from Virginia Beach back to his home in Arlington, Texas. At this point he was starting to get fed up with the high doses of prescription medications his doctors had him taking. He didn't feel like the VA was helping him at all with his health issues: "They'd rather just send me a bunch of pills in the mail and tell me to take them." Then, in the spring of 2014, he heard about Dr. Sue Sisley and her research project on veterans and PTSD and decided to start considering other options for both his pain and his PTSD. He had never been to Colorado before, but he knew about the availability of a variety of medical cannabis in the state. So in 2014 he "packed up [his] whole life in a U-Haul truck and moved up here without ever having set foot in the state." As with so many others, Zach soon found the relief he was looking for with marijuana. He found that cannabis was very therapeutic and helped him to wean himself off of his mass doses of pharmaceuticals. He now uses daily cannabis oil for pain relief and for the stress and anxiety associated with PTSD. Like many other medical refugees, Zach has no regrets although the move had its challenges for him. He has since been involved in veteran activism in the state, including the fight to have PTSD added as a qualifying medical condition.

Veterans like Zach Phillips, Matt Kahl, and Rocky Hall might move to Colorado for access to cannabis, but they also end up finding community. In many cases this community leads to activism, both on the local and the national level. National organizations like Weed for Warriors have been leading the way in publicizing the health problems veterans in this nation face and their need for access to legal cannabis. This organization has chapters across the U.S. and organizes protests and rallies to bring attention to issues of PTSD, suicide, and overprescription in the veteran community. Past protests have included "smoke-ins" and "die-ins" in Washington, D.C., as well as dumping mass amounts of prescription pill bottles in front of the White House.[29] Such actions have brought media and public attention to the plight being faced by veterans and to the call for legal medical marijuana. Many veterans are involved with organizations that, in addition to political protests, help to educate other veterans about cannabis. An organization called Grow for Vets, which has chapters in most legal states, is a nonprofit whose mission is to "connect Veterans with the knowledge and resources necessary to obtain or grow their own cannabis for the treatment of their medical conditions."[30] The national nonprofit Veteran's Cannabis Project aims to bring together different organizations and "to foster an environment that is politically and legally favorable to US military veterans using medical marijuana to address service-related health challenges that prevent them from living the high quality of life that they have earned."[31]

In Colorado, not only are many veteran medical refugees involved in these national advocacy efforts but they also helped to spearhead one of the most effective cannabis policy changes in recent times. Advocates have been trying for years to get PTSD listed as a qualifying condition for medical marijuana, and veterans have taken a leading role in that fight. When medical marijuana was first legalized in Colorado back in the year 2000 there were eight qualifying conditions (AIDS/HIV, glaucoma, cachexia, persistent muscle spasms, cancer, seizures, severe nausea, and severe pain), none of which were psychological conditions.[32] Many patients had been forced to lie, saying they had "chronic severe pain" in order to qualify for medical marijuana, or after 2012 to use much-higher-priced recreational marijuana without a doctor's guidance. The legal fight to add PTSD to the qualifying conditions list started in 2010 when Brian Vicente, a Denver lawyer, along with a group of veterans, presented Colorado's chief medical officer at the time, Ned Colange, with a petition. Later that year the board of health rejected the petition, and it would go on to reject three more petitions in the following years.[33]

The last rejection by the board of health occurred in 2015 after a heated hearing during which dozens of constituents testified in favor of adding PTSD, including researcher Dr. Sue Sisley, multiple veterans with PTSD, including Matt Kahl, and medical doctors like Dr. Joe Cohen. Despite a recommendation from the state's Medical Marijuana Scientific Advisory Counsel, including Colorado chief medical officer Larry Wolk, that PTSD be added to the list of conditions, the board voted 6–2 against adding the disorder, saying they needed "more concrete evidence."[34] At this point advocates decided they needed another tactic, and five PTSD patients, including Matt Kahl, along with marijuana lawyer Bob Hoban, "sued the board and the Colorado Department of Public Health and Environment over its decision."[35] Meanwhile, advocates also decided to try a route that had previously been attempted in 2014—introducing a bill in the Colorado legislature. Although the bill fell short that session they were confident they might have greater support this time. In the summer of 2016 patient advocacy groups presented their case to the legislature's interim committee on marijuana. State senator Irene Aguilar was swayed by their presentations, along with the fact that the CDPHE supported adding the condition, and cosponsored SB17–017 late that year. In 2017 the bill passed through the legislature, and Governor Hickenlooper signed it into law on June 5, making Colorado the 23rd state or U.S. territory to allow medical cannabis for PTSD.[36]

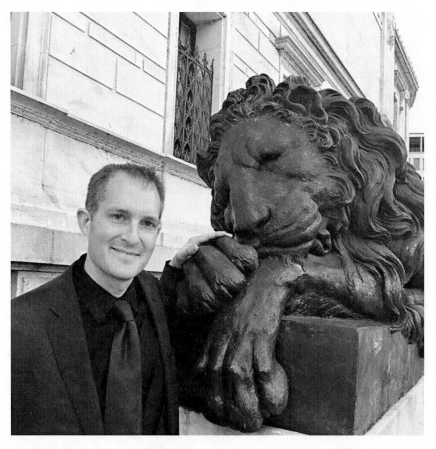

After finding success with using cannabis for his PTSD, army veteran Matt Kahl became an advocate for the drug, working to get PTSD added to the list of qualifying conditions in Colorado (courtesy Matt Kahl).

While veterans who live in or move to Colorado are now able to use medical marijuana for PTSD, chronic pain, and other medical conditions and often find a supportive community in which to do so, the same cannot be said for vets in many other parts of the country. One such veteran, Kris Lewandowski, attempted to use cannabis for his PTSD in the state of Oklahoma and found himself in deep trouble with law enforcement. Kris, who graduated from high school and community college in Colorado, decided to enlist in the Marines in 2005. He had originally wanted to be a police officer, but after 9/11 occurred and the war in the Middle East began he decided he wanted to serve his country in Iraq and deployed there shortly after enlisting. Kris married his wife, Whitney, in 2010 and went on to serve two more tours overseas. During that time he suffered injuries to his shoulder and back and began to develop PTSD. After his return to the states Kris, like so many other vets, was prescribed a multitude of pharmaceuticals for his pain and worsening mental condition. Nothing seemed to help, however, and he was medically retired and honorably discharged.[37]

Around this time, the Lewandowskis' first child was born and the family moved to Ft. Sill in Lawton, Oklahoma, where Kris worked as an instructor while awaiting his retirement processing. The PTSD and the various pharmaceuticals he was on began to really affect his mental health. He recalls, "The pills were making things worse, it wasn't making it better. I was sad, I was mad, and the PTSD and pain were still there…. The PTSD and varying pharmaceuticals to treat it were stealing my soul. Stress was intolerable, life wasn't worth living, I was fighting for my life, I wanted to die, and taking the pills the doctors gave me didn't stop that feeling, they made it worse."[38] Knowing he needed to make a change, especially for his wife and two children (their second child was born in Oklahoma), Kris began to wean himself off of his prescriptions and looked into natural treatments for his PTSD. One vet after another recommended the same thing to Kris: marijuana.

So, in June 2014, Kris started growing a few marijuana plants, six to be exact, just enough to treat his PTSD symptoms. Meanwhile, he was trying to wean himself off of his pharmaceuticals. His untreated PTSD and opiate withdrawal and his wife's postpartum state led to frequent arguments. One night she made a domestic disturbance call, and when the police showed up at the house they found the six plants. They told Whitney that if she did not file a domestic violence charge against him (he had been found in the kitchen with a knife), they would charge her for the plants as well, and they would lose custody of their two young sons. Whitney now says, however, that she never felt in danger. She told *Truth in Media*, "They're trying to use me as a victim and to make it look worse on his case. My husband has absolutely never laid his hands on me ever. He is not an abusive man, ever … quite the opposite. He is extremely doting."[39]

While six plants being grown for medical use would not be a serious issue in most states, Oklahoma's marijuana laws at the time were some of the strictest in the country. The local media called the discovery of the plants a "major pot bust," and Sheriff Kenny Stradley told the local ABC affiliate, KSWO-TV, "When we get there and we find out we have marijuana there that's being grown, it seems to get worse. And then with children present this is a bad situation gone worse for the whole entire family."[40] Even though the entire weight of the marijuana found on the small plants was less than one ounce, Kris was charged with felony marijuana cultivation, which carries a maximum sentence of life in prison in the state of Oklahoma. Kris's first lawyer convinced him to take a plea deal to avoid the longest sentence, but it meant being labeled a felon and he soon realized his mistake. He went back to court in October 2016 to plead his case and was able to overturn the plea deal. He then returned to court in May 2017 to be sentenced on his charges. Perhaps because of the outpouring of support from around the country, the sentencing went well. Kris pleaded guilty to a deferred felony charge for marijuana cultivation, "meaning that if he does not violate the law during a five-year probation period, no felony will be placed on his record."[41]

Kris Lewandowski, his wife, Whitney, and their three children now live in their home state of California. Kris is involved with Weed for Warriors and other marijuana advocacy groups for vets and is successfully using cannabis to treat his PTSD, which is so severe he is classified as 100 percent disabled by the military. While his story has a happy ending, no one, especially a ten-year combat veteran who saw three tours of duty, should have to face those sorts of legal repercussions for attempting to treat their medical conditions with a plant that is legal for use in over half the states in the country.

Conclusion:
Why Federal Policy
Must Change

It is April 7, 2017. Shona Banda sits in a court in Garden City, Kansas, for arraignment and a pretrial conference. She pleads not guilty to five felony counts of possession of marijuana with intent to distribute, manufacturing THC oil from cannabis, two counts of possession of drug paraphernalia, and one count of child endangerment.[1] But Shona is not a dangerous cartel leader or drug dealer. She is a middle-aged mom who uses marijuana oil to treat her chronic Crohn's disease. Although at the time of her arrest medical marijuana in some form was legal in the majority of states, she lives in a state where it is still completely prohibited. She is facing harsh penalties.

Shona Banda has lived with the pain and suffering of Crohn's disease since 2002. She has undergone 15 surgeries for the condition, including having parts of her intestines removed and undergoing a complete hysterectomy at the age of 29 because of scar tissue. Like most Crohn's sufferers, she has also tried a multitude of powerful pharmaceuticals, none of which were effective. By the time Shona reached her early 30s, doctors told her that there was nothing else they could do and they prescribed her the narcotic fentanyl to "ease her passing."[2] At this time she was smoking marijuana to help with pain and stress, but it did not cure the symptoms of her Crohn's. She told the *Washington Post*, "I spent years raising my children from a couch, not being able to move much. I wasn't able to be a proper mother when I was sick."[3] Then she heard about the healing properties of cannabis oil and gave it a try. In an interview with radio host Ben Swann, Banda recalled how quickly the oil worked: "I went from feeling

... the pain from dying to literally waking up on day three knowing that I was going to live long enough to see my grandkids someday."[4]

Because of the prohibition in Kansas on medical marijuana Shona tried twice to move to Colorado, but both times she had to return to Kansas for financial reasons. Eventually she started travelling to Colorado to buy marijuana and brought it back to Kansas to make her medicinal oil. Then one day in 2015 her 11-year-old son spoke up about her use of marijuana at a school anti-drug presentation. That same day, school officials called the police and child protective services.[5] The Garden City police raided Shona's residence and "approximately 500 grams of suspected marijuana, multiple marijuana smoking pipes, three 'vaporizers' that were actively manufacturing cannabis oil and multiple other items related to packaging and ingestion of marijuana were seized from the residence."[6] Shona was arrested and charged, and her son was taken away by child protective services and placed first with his father then with the state and then back with his father.[7]

For using a medicine that is completely legal just one state to the west, Shona Banda lost both her child and her access to lifesaving medicine and faced up to 30 years in jail. But she continued to fight back. She filed a lawsuit in federal court in March of 2016 that named the Garden City Police Department, Garden City USD 456, and the State of Kansas, among others, and "alleged that her rights to use cannabis for medicinal purposes and to maintain custody of her son had been violated." The lawsuit was dismissed by a federal judge.[8] The following year, at her April arraignment, Shona pleaded not guilty to all charges and also had two medical doctors testify via telecommunications devices to be allowed as expert witnesses in her upcoming trial. Both doctors are experts in cannabinoids and cannabis-based medicine and have served as expert witnesses in various other trials. Shona reached a plea deal in August 2017, pleading no contest to "possession of drug paraphernalia with intent to manufacture, a felony." In exchange, the county attorney's office agreed to dismiss several other charges and support probation terms that allowed her to leave the state. She then moved to Washington state to be able to use her medicine legally while she awaited sentencing.[9] Fortunately for the sake of her health, in October of that same year she was sentenced to 12 months of probation, which she would be allowed to serve from Washington with check-ins via mail.[10]

Shona Banda is not the only medical marijuana user who has been prosecuted and had their child taken away in the state of Kansas. In 2015 Raymond Schwab, a navy Gulf War veteran who worked for Veterans Affairs, requested a transfer to Colorado so that he could start growing marijuana for his own and other veterans' medical use.[11] Schwab, who suffers from severe PTSD, was already a licensed medical user in Colorado and had been using cannabis to control his symptoms for years.[12] In fact, Schwab says that he suffered from mental issues (stemming from his PTSD) for a long time, and the pharmaceuticals prescribed for his condition led to opiate and, later, heroin addiction. Cannabis helped him to get off of heroin and "is the only medication that helps with his anxiety, depression and physical pain."[13] Because he was forced to use the drug illegally in Kansas, he made the decision to move his family to Colorado. However, when he and his wife took a short trip to Colorado to scout a place to live, they left their five children (ages 5, 7, 11, 13, and 16) with relatives.[14] One of those relatives reported his children as "abandoned," and they were subsequently seized by the state. While the family had minor scrapes with the law in the past, Schwab says, "None of those things were in the state's allegation ... but marijuana was."[15]

Raymond and his wife, Amelia, spent over two years desperately trying to get their kids back. They moved to Colorado to access cannabis medicine, but they return to Kansas regularly. While the Kansas Department of Children and Families (DCF) said "children are not removed from the home for [parental] marijuana use alone," claims of "emotional abuse" have been found to be unsubstantiated.[16] In fact, included in police evidence against the Schwabs is a "screenshot of Schwab's recent Facebook post, where he discusses moving to Colorado to start a marijuana business."[17] Additionally, in a court hearing in October 2017, the judge asked that the couple submit to urinalysis and told them they would need to be free of marijuana in their systems before being allowed to visit with their children—this, despite the fact that Amelia and Raymond have since moved to Colorado, where both have medical cards for marijuana.[18] As the local news reported, the judge in the case, John Bosch, "was skeptical of the Schwab's use of marijuana."[19] After that, Raymond Schwab went on a hunger strike and the couple took their case to court. Finally, in November 2017, a Kansas judge ruled that the children could go to live with their parents in Colorado at the end of that year.[20]

Unfortunately, it is not uncommon in certain parts of the country for parents to lose custody of their children due to marijuana use. Jennifer Ani, a renowned family law attorney in California, says that she sees around five cases like that of the Schwabs every month and that 95 percent of the time, she believes, "the child was in no reasonable danger."[21] The discrepancies between federal law, legal states' policies, and prohibition states' laws have led to "a growing gap between what's legal and what raises red flags for child-protection agencies."[22] The U.S. Department of Health and Human Services has a pamphlet entitled "Parental Drug Use as Child Abuse," which states "exposing children to the manufacture, possession, or distribution of illegal drugs is considered child endangerment in 11 States [including Kansas]."[23] Because marijuana is still a federally illegal drug, using the drug in a child's presence, even in a legal state, could thus be construed as child abuse. The Family Law and Cannabis Alliance, a Massachusetts-based group formed in 2013 to help parents in marijuana-related child-welfare and custody disputes, says it "assisted 200 families nationwide" in 2014.[24] Additionally, public defenders in Colorado who represent clients in family and juvenile court estimate that about "one-sixth of their cases involve marijuana."[25] Across the country, families are still being torn apart by the antiquated war on marijuana.

Additionally, although cannabis laws are changing at an ever-increasing pace, arrests for marijuana possession remain high. In 2016 the *New York Times* reported on a study that found that, nationwide, arrests for possession of small amounts of marijuana surpassed arrests for all violent crimes in the previous year. The study, released by the American Civil Liberties Union and Human Rights Watch, found that there were 574,641 arrests for possession of small amounts of cannabis (intended for personal use) in 2015, which amounts to around one arrest every minute.[26] Even one hundred years after the start of the war on marijuana in the United States, and despite much legal progress, the injustices that underpin cannabis prohibition remain.

The situation is at its worst in a handful of states that still enforce draconian marijuana laws and penalties. In 2015 over half of the drug arrests in Texas were for marijuana, and 97 percent of those were for possession of two ounces or less.[27] Texas state representative and former attorney Joe Moody says that he has seen young lives destroyed because of the penalties that go along with these possession arrests. He explained: "If they are convicted of that offence you are looking at if you had financial aid grants those could be off the table for you, federal student aid is definitely off the table, getting a job is going to be extremely difficult because those criminal background checks are going to show up. Renting an apartment. Anything a young person is needing to be doing to kind of get on their feet to get their life going, all those things can be derailed by a minor conviction."[28] Although in Colorado possession is legal and in many states it is not a criminal offense, in states like Texas possession of a few joints could end up ruining someone's life.

That is exactly what happened in 2010 to Bernard Noble, a 45-year-old trucker and father of seven children who had two previous nonviolent offenses (for drug possession). Noble was stopped by police on a street in New Orleans and arrested for having two joints in his pocket. Due to Louisiana's hard-line stance on drug possession, Noble was sentenced to 13.3 years in prison without the possibility of parole. This sentence not only takes Bernard Noble away from his children until they are grown but Louisiana also loses a productive member of society and "Mr. Noble's prison sentence for possessing two joints will cost Louisiana taxpayers nearly one-quarter of a million dollars."[29] As Jesse Wegman writes in a *New York Times* op-ed, these long, costly prison sentences are only part of the story. Drug convictions affect those who are arrested in multiple ways, from student loans to housing to jobs. Wegman asserts, "The hundreds of thousands of people who are arrested each year but do not go to jail also suffer; their arrests stay on their records for years, crippling their prospects for jobs, loans, housing and benefits."

As long as marijuana remains an illegal Schedule I drug at the federal level, millions of users around the United States will continue to suffer negative consequences. Patients in dozens of states where the full-plant medicine is illegal or unavailable will have to make the choice to move to a state like Colorado—with better, safer access—or remain at home. Those who have to stay will need to choose between using an unregulated product (if they can access it) with possible legal repercussions or pass up a treatment that could be lifesaving. And federal prohibition will continue to create social justice issues—disproportionately affecting people of color and lower economic classes. It is obviously more difficult to move across the country to seek cannabis treatment without sufficient funds or the ability to relocate one's job.

In addition to facing greater financial barriers to moving to another state, patients of lower economic status who stay in prohibition states (or states with less-progressive medical marijuana laws) and pursue treatments are more likely to face legal repercussions. This is especially true for black and Hispanic users. As seen by the stories of Shona Banda and other patients, legalization in many states has not stopped arrests for marijuana in other parts of the country. In fact, an FBI report released in September 2018 showed that marijuana arrests actually increased in 2017, with 659,700 arrests, or "one marijuana bust roughly every 48 seconds."[30] Marijuana continues to constitute nearly half of all drug arrests, and a full 90.8 percent of those charged with marijuana law violations in 2017 were arrested for possession only.[31] Additionally, despite multiple surveys showing similar rates of use among different races, arrest rates continue to be disproportionate for blacks and Hispanics as compared to whites. A 2015 study in New Jersey showed that black residents of certain cities were 2.6 to 9.6 times more likely to be arrested for low-level marijuana offences.[32] More recently, in New York City, where medical marijuana is legal and usage is widespread, roughly 89 percent of the 4,000 people arrested for possession in the first three months of 2018 were black or Hispanic.[33] The *New York Times* reports that in Manhattan blacks are 15 times more likely than whites to be arrested for marijuana. Despite looser marijuana laws and declining crime rates, the marijuana arrest rates for blacks and Hispanics have remained roughly the same for decades.[34]

Besides facing more arrest risks, people of color and lower income individuals also face a higher probability of having their children taken away as a result of those individuals consuming marijuana or treating their sick children with marijuana. Not only do states have a variety of different laws around medical cannabis but states also have different statutes regarding what constitutes child abuse and neglect. In California the government must prove "actual harm" in order to take custody of a child, whereas New York does not require any proof of harm.[35] Such varying regulations leave much room for the individual discretion (and biases) of social workers, judges, and police. In New York City "lawyers say the drug plays a role in perpetuating racial and class disparities in the city's foster care system," where approximately 93 percent of the 11,000 foster children in the city are Hispanic or black. If a parent tests positive for marijuana they are often required to attend drug counseling before they are allowed to reunite with their child. For low income parents such stipulations can be particularly difficult. As Emma Ketteringham, a family defense attorney in New York, says, "Parents of privilege talk openly about their use of marijuana. They have absolutely no idea that some parents have to visit their children in an agency because they continue to test positive for marijuana."[36] With a medley of state and county laws, biased perspectives on marijuana, race, or poverty can lead to negative impacts on parents who use medical marijuana, and their children.

Despite the majority of states legalizing either medical or full adult use of cannabis, the federal gov-

Timeline of marijuana legalization in the U.S. (Third Way).

STATE MARIJUANA LEGALIZATION TIMELINE

YEAR	MEDICAL	RECREATIONAL
1996	California	
1997		
1998	Alaska Oregon Washington	
1999	Maine	
2000	Colorado Hawaii Nevada	
2001		
2002		
2003		
2004	Montana Vermont	
2005		
2006	Rhode Island	
2007	New Mexico	
2008	Michigan	
2009		
2010	Arizona New Mexico New Jersey Washington, D.C.	
2011	Delaware	
2012	Connecticut Massachusetts	Colorado Washington
2013	Illinois New Hampshire	
2014	Maryland Minnesota New York	Alaska Oregon Washington, D.C.
2015		
2016	Arkansas Florida North Dakota Ohio Pennsylvania	California Maine Massachusetts Nevada Vermont
2017	West Virginia	
2018	Missouri Oklahoma Utah	Michigan

ernment remains mired in the drug war attitudes of the 20th century. Even as more and more people discover the healing benefits of cannabis, the DEA refuses to de-schedule or even re-schedule the drug from its current Schedule I abode. As my multiple interviews and research demonstrate, these outdated policies have real life and death consequences for people throughout the country: Angela Kastner, a grandmother with terminal cancer who was jailed in Kansas in 2017 for driving with THC in her system, THC that she was prescribed by her doctor for her chemotherapy-induced nausea[37]; Larry Burgess, a Kansas man facing several felony charges related to his use of cannabis oil for his seizures (when he was arrested in 2017 and not allowed access to his cannabis medicine he seized that night and had to be taken to the hospital)[38]; Maria Green, a California mom and medicinal marijuana caregiver who lost custody of her 6-month-old child because she was growing cannabis for her epileptic husband.[39] For every patient who has found healing with cannabis or every person who has run afoul of the law in the attempt for healing there are hundreds, if not thousands, who will never know if this medicine would work for them because they will never have the chance to try it.

In a time of rapidly changing drug laws and political uncertainty, Colorado has provided thousands of patients with access to life-altering medicinal cannabis. However, not everyone who needs marijuana can relocate to Colorado or another legal state to access the drug, and these states certainly could not absorb all of those people even if the people could move. While Colorado's successful "experiment" with legal marijuana can serve as a template for the rest of the nation and the world, as can the lessons learned from our community of medical marijuana refugees, we need to make the term "medical refugee" unnecessary. Nobody should have to flee a war, certainly not a war on the very medicine that could save their life. It's time to end the destructive war on marijuana and the people who use it and provide access to this medicine for those who need it across the entire nation. Colorado has proven that the drug is beneficial and can be regulated effectively. Let's not wait any longer to de-schedule at the federal level. Thousands of patients are already running out of time.

Epilogue:
What Now?

The world of cannabis is changing at a blistering pace. It is almost impossible to keep up with legal changes, and the cannabis industry and scientific research is snowballing. Since I began research for this book in 2015, seven states—California, Nevada, Maine, Massachusetts, Vermont, Michigan, and Illinois—have passed full adult legalization of marijuana. Ten more states (Pennsylvania, Ohio, Arkansas, Florida, North Dakota, West Virginia, Oklahoma, Maryland, Utah, and Missouri) have passed comprehensive medical marijuana policies (see Appendix A for more detailed information on state laws including those that are still pending). Internationally, laws still lag behind individual states in the U.S., but Canada did enact full legalization for adults in 2018.

In the past few years several states have also passed less effective CBD-only policies in an attempt to assuage their constituents' desire for medical cannabis. However, patients in these states often need more complete cannabis therapy, and even if CBD oil could help them many have trouble accessing the medicine. The issue is further complicated by the federal government's complex and contradictory stance on the drug, or as Dr. Jamie Corroon and Rod Kight write for Project CBD, "cannabis law is a lot wackier than the weed."[1] First, CBD's legality depends on whether it is derived from hemp (cannabis that contains less than .3 percent THC) or marijuana (cannabis with higher than .3 percent THC).[2] Many say that CBD that comes from hemp is legal under federal law due to the 2018 Farm Bill, which legalized industrial hemp. However, the Farm Bill legalized hemp cultivation only under restricted circumstances. In addition to requiring that industrialized hemp contain less than .3 percent THC, the new Farm Bill requires that states and the

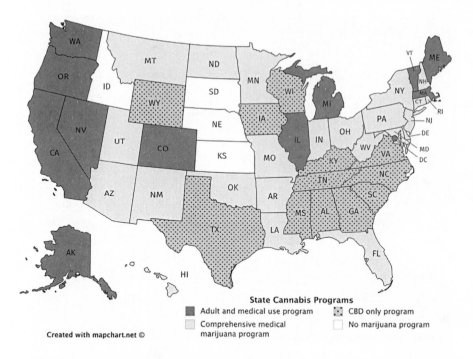

State Cannabis Programs

- Adult and medical use program
- Comprehensive medical marijuana program
- CBD only program
- No marijuana program

Created with mapchart.net ©

Map of the United States showing various degrees of cannabis legalization by state (National Conference of State Legislatures).

federal government share regulatory powers over the industry.[3] According to section 10113 of the bill, "state departments of agriculture must consult with the state's governor and chief law enforcement officer to devise a plan that must be submitted to the Secretary of USDA. A state's plan to license and regulate hemp can only commence once the Secretary of USDA approves that state's plan."[4] Finally, the bill outlines which actions are considered federal violations (including unregulated growing) and the possible punishments for such violations, some of which are even felonies. Thus, as the Brookings Institute's John Hudak notes, although the Farm Bill does legalize hemp "it doesn't create a system in which people can grow it as freely as they can grow tomatoes or basil. This will be a highly regulated crop in the United States for both personal and industrial production."[5]

To add to the confusion, although the 2018 Farm Bill does remove hemp-derived CBD from Schedule I status, it does not legalize CBD generally. CBD is exempted from the Controlled Substances Act only if the hemp it is derived from is produced in "a manner consistent with the Farm Bill, associated federal regulations, associated state regulations, and by a licensed grower."[6] The one exception is pharmaceutical-grade CBD products approved by the FDA, but so far only one product, GW Pharma's Epidiolex, has been approved.[7] Additionally, CBD in food and beverage products is never legal according to the FDA because CBD has never been approved for that purpose.[8] Of course, these products continue to be sold in many states but are still illegal at the federal level.

While lack of legal consistency adds to the confusion for cannabis patients nationwide, those in legal states worry about marijuana's future nationwide due to a volatile political climate. Although Donald Trump expressed support for medical marijuana during his campaign, his appointment of conservative lawyer Jeff Sessions as attorney general had many fearing for the legal future of medical cannabis. In May of 2017 Sessions asked Congress to undo the Rohrabacher-Farr amendment, a move that would remove "federal medical-marijuana protections that have been in place since 2014."[9] Although Sessions did not have much support in Congress, his anti-cannabis stance was clear. As a senator he had compared marijuana to heroin and was one of the most avowed opponents of legalization. In May of 2017 he also convened a Justice Department task force to review marijuana policies, a task force that included several anti-marijuana members. While the task force largely recommended for the status quo in its July 2017 report, Sessions continued to consider ways to overturn pro-cannabis regulations.[10] Fortunately for legal cannabis proponents, Sessions was forced to resign by Trump in November of 2018.[11] However, in December 2018 Trump announced his intention to nominate William Barr as his new attorney general. This news was met with concern by cannabis advocates and industry groups alike. The National Organization for the Reform of Marijuana Laws voiced its trepidation over his possible nomination, since his support of the war on drugs could leave the future of legal cannabis uncertain.[12]

Even amid political concerns about possible crackdowns, however, national attitudes toward cannabis are becoming more positive, states continue to legalize, and the industry is growing at a record-breaking pace. A 2017 Marist University survey found that marijuana use "has gone mainstream." The survey found that nearly 55 million American adults currently use marijuana and that most Americans think smoking marijuana is "socially acceptable, and the vast majority believe that marijuana use is less risky than use of alcohol, tobacco or painkillers (72 percent believe alcohol use is riskier, 78 percent think tobacco use is riskier, and 67 percent said that prescription painkiller use is riskier than use of cannabis)."[13] Perhaps most important for medical patients, a Quinnipiac poll released in August 2017 found support for medical marijuana at an all-time high, with 94 percent of Americans agreeing that the U.S. should allow "adults to legally use marijuana for medical purposes if their doctor prescribes it."[14] These statistics explain the liberalization of marijuana laws at the state level and also show that the federal government may be out of step with the mainstream of America when it comes to this particular drug.

The marijuana business is also changing and growing rapidly, not only with the industrial hemp industry poised to flourish in the coming years but also with medical and recreational markets increasing exponentially. In June 2017 the National Association of Cannabis Businesses (NACB) launched as the "first self-regulatory organization of the industry."[15] The organization formed in order to "be ready" for federal legalization and put forth a plan to "develop and enforce national standards that will increase compliance and transparency, spur growth, and shape future federal regulations."[16] Such a move is no surprise in an industry that grew 30 percent throughout North America in 2016, totaling $6.7 billion in sales. In the states of Colorado, Washington, and Oregon (which have established cannabis industries), sales jumped 62 percent from 2015 to 2016.[17] *Forbes* writer Debra Borchardt notes, "To put this in perspective, this industry growth is larger and faster than even the dot-com era. During that time, GDP grew at a blistering pace of 22%. Thirty percent is an astounding number especially when you consider that the industry is in early stages."[18] Various analytic firms have projected sales topping $20 billion by 2021 and $24 billion by 2025, with the state of California alone projected to have more than $6.5 billion in sales by the time its industry becomes fully operational.[19] Perhaps most important to the medical cannabis industry, which resides in medical and legal limbo, is a study from New Frontier Data hypothesizing that medical marijuana could siphon $4 billion from pharmaceutical sales annually.[20]

While laws, attitudes, and the cannabis industry continue to evolve rapidly, less has changed for medical marijuana refugees, especially as the drug remains federally prohibited and state laws are still inconsistent. Many patients and their families continue to move to legal states, including Colorado, in search of better access to their medicine. While no specific statistics exist to determine how many people are moving to Colorado specifically to access cannabis, American Medical Refugees continues to grow and to field dozens of requests from refugees and potential refugees every week. Of the families I interviewed for this book, only one has returned to their home state due to legal changes around medical cannabis there. All of the others remain in Colorado for the medical advantages.

The one family that was able to return home is the Turners—Wendy and Tommy, and their son, Coltyn, who continues to use cannabis for his Crohn's disease. They were able to return to their home in southern Illinois after the state legalized medical cannabis and set up a functioning dispensary system. Although the former governor approved a pilot program in 2013, it wasn't until the current governor signed an extension bill in 2016 that the program really became established.[21] Nevertheless, "Illinois' program remains one of the most restrictive in the nation," and the Turners waited until Coltyn was 18 before making the move.[22] They returned to Illinois in the summer of 2018, and within a couple of months Coltyn had his medical card and was able to start accessing his medicine.

Although legalization opened up an avenue for the Turners to return home, most patients decide to remain in their new state after moving for marijuana. The Hilterbrans, whose son Austin has Dravet's syndrome, decided to put down roots in Colorado and recently purchased 35 acres for a hemp and organic medicinals farm. Austin has turned 17, outliving the doctors' prognosis by more than 3 years. Cannabis continues to work for him, as he goes weeks and sometimes months with no seizures at all. Additionally, he is off of all the pharmaceuticals that were causing his organs to shut down and tests show that there is no longer any notable damage to his kidneys or liver. Jason and Amy's two younger sons both have had seizures, but the couple decided to forego pharmaceuticals altogether and start treatment right away with cannabis. Amy reports that this treatment has been highly successful for them, with no further seizures at all after cannabis.

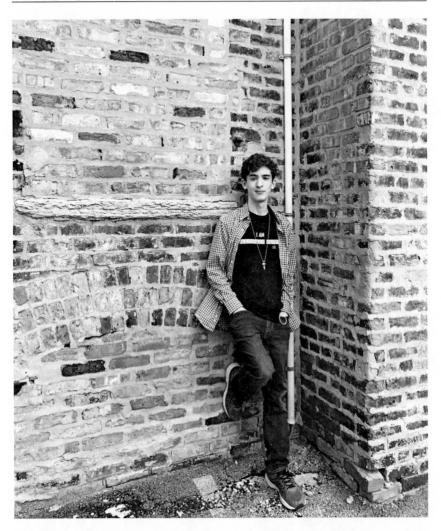

After his home state of Illinois legalized medical marijuana and he turned 18, Coltyn Turner returned to the state where he now lives and continues to advocate for marijuana (courtesy Wendy Turner).

Other families and patients profiled in this book also remain in Colorado and continue to see success with cannabis medicine. Many, like the Domers from North Carolina and the Roots from Florida, cannot return home because full-spectrum medical cannabis is not available in their home states. Others, like the Sanchezes, stay because they have forged a new home in Colorado, supported by the community they have found here. Regardless of their reasons for staying, most continue to see success with their cannabis treatment. Novaleigh Harris, who was born missing part of her brain, has now far surpassed the expectations of her doctors back in Texas. Since moving to Colorado with her parents, Joseph Harris and Barbara Bunker, Novaleigh's seizures are much better controlled and she has surpassed all her doctor's predictions. Jackson Stormes is also doing well; he was weaned off of almost all of his pharmaceuticals with the help of cannabis and then no longer needed to use marijuana. Now his condition is controlled with a minimal number of drugs and he has been able to travel to the beach and to Disney World with his mother, Jennie Stormes. Little Landon Riddle, whose cancer went into remission after he moved with his mother, Sierra Riddle, to Colorado for treatment with cannabis, continues to be cancer free. He is now a healthy nine-year-old.

Despite the success stories of so many medical marijuana refugees and despite the incredible gains in legislation and research around the country, the future of marijuana in medicine remains uncertain. Without federal re-scheduling or de-scheduling, the legal status of cannabis will continue to vary wildly, with a hodgepodge of regulations from state to state and researchers struggling to conduct federally recognized clinical trials. If the stories of the first wave of medical refugees can teach us anything, it's that this drug has incredible potential and that we need change at the federal level. Until then, the only thing certain about the future of medical marijuana is uncertainty.

University of Colorado School of Medicine Guidelines for Human Subject Research Involving Cannabis as of February 2016

For all studies:

- Cannot accept funding for research from cannabis industry.

For observational studies:

- Can survey or evaluate subjects who are already using drug for medical or recreational purposes (e.g., can ask subject to come in for a blood draw one hour after taking drug).
- Should obtain federal Certificate of Confidentiality for the study. Cannot subsidize the purchase of the cannabis products.
- Cannot pay subjects to participate in the study.
- Cannot bring to campus cannabis products to test level of cannabinoids (e.g., from grower or retailer).
- Cannot advise or prescribe to start taking the drug or manage it in any way.
- Cannot dictate when the drug is to be given (e.g., specific times to enable pharmacokinetic studies).
- Cannot ask users to stop cannabis use to be eligible to participate in a study (e.g., no baseline studies).
- Cannot ask to stop using drug for a washout period.
- Cannot have subjects smoke or ingest drug anywhere on campus before being interviewed or evaluated for research.
- Cannot advise or prescribe to start taking the drug.

- Cannot move people higher on waiting list for a certain product at the dispensary if they agree to participate in a study.

For interventional studies (including animal studies):

- Must be conducted under an IND from the FDA.
- Can use only cannabis purchased from NIDA or a cannabis-derived product that has an FDA record (FDA approved or under IND).
- Must apply for a DEA researcher registration.
- Cannot add marijuana to clinical DEA license.
- Must use specifically designed and dedicated locations for storage and administration of the drug.
- Must post study on ClinicalTrials.gov posting as Applicable Clinical Trial.
- Study results need to be posted no later than 12 months after the final collection of the primary outcome data.

DEA = Drug Enforcement Agency; FDA = Food and Drug Administration; IND = investigational new drug; NIDA = National Institute on Drug Abuse.

*From Edward Hoffenberg et al., "Cannabis and Pediatric Inflammatory Bowel Disease."

APPENDIX B

Resources

Support Groups for Patients

American Alliance for Medical Cannabis (AAMC)
www.letfreedomgrow.com
Founded in 2001, AAMC is a coalition of health professionals, patients, caregivers, community members, and experts in the field of cannabis. Their mission is patient advocacy, patient rights, and support.

Americans for Safe Access
https://www.safeaccessnow.org/
The mission of this organization is to ensure safe and legal access to marijuana for therapeutic use and research. Their website is incredibly comprehensive, with patient resources, legal information, news and advocacy reports.

American Medical Refugees
Contact: AmericanMedicalRefugees@yahoo.com
Based in Colorado, this group provides resources for those who have had to relocate in order to access medical cannabis for themselves or a family member. They have a Facebook group that can be joined with moderator permission. They also hold various events for families in Colorado and provide a venue for marijuana refugees to communicate, share their stories, and gain access to information.

Cannabis Patients Alliance
https://cannabispatientsalliance.org/
Founded by Coloradan Teri Robnett, Cannabis Patients Alliance "is an alliance of patients, families, organizations, businesses, advocates, activists and other supporters who work together to protect and advance

the rights of patients who choose to use medical cannabis (marijuana) to treat whatever their condition may be." Their website contains news and policy information as well as an extensive list of patient resources.

Patients Out of Time
http://www.medicalcannabis.com/
This Virginia-based nonprofit aims "to educate all disciplines of health care professionals; their specialty and professional organizations; the legal profession; and the public at large, about medical cannabis (marijuana)." Their website contains links for patients and medical professionals as well as scientific and useful information about cannabis.

United Patients Group
https://unitedpatientsgroup.com/
This California organization, although somewhat commercial, nevertheless has a comprehensive website with information for patients and health care workers. They also organize educational conferences on medical cannabis.

Veterans Groups

HeroGrown
https://herogrown.org/
Formerly known as Grow for Vets USA, this group provides education and awareness about medical marijuana, advocates for legal change, and provides CBD products free of charge to thousands of needy veterans and first responders.

Veterans Cannabis Coalition
https://www.veteranscannacoalition.org/
This organization "is dedicated to ensuring that veterans have access to the medicine they need without fear or stigmatization. We are focused on engaging stakeholders, educating policymakers and the public, and advocating for fair and equitable cannabis laws."

Veterans Cannabis Group
http://www.veteranscannabisgroup.com/
Veterans Cannabis Groups is an educational resource for veterans and their families. They hold regular conference calls for members.

Veterans Cannabis Project (VCP)
https://www.vetscp.org/
VCG advocates for veterans' rights to access legal and safe medical cannabis, educates them on their health options, and supports cannabis research.

Weed for Warriors
https://www.wfwproject.org/
This California-based organization also has chapters across the country to bring veterans together for education and advocacy about medical cannabis.

Political Advocacy

Americans for Safe Access (ASA)
https://www.safeaccessnow.org/about_asa
Founded in 2002, ASA's mission is "to ensure safe and legal access to cannabis (marijuana) for therapeutic use and research." Their website contains a large quantity of resources for patients, medical professionals, legislators, information on laws and rights, along with links to publications and news.

Drug Policy Alliance
http://www.drugpolicy.org/
The Drug Policy Alliance is the largest drug policy reform organization in the United States. While they work toward all types of drug policy reform for all drugs, including harm reduction policies, their website has information on marijuana and marijuana policy reform campaigns.

Marijuana Policy Project
https://www.mpp.org/
The Marijuana Policy Project focuses on changing marijuana policy and public opinion around the drug. Their mission is to "increase public support for non-punitive, non-coercive marijuana policies. Identify and activate supporters of non-punitive, non-coercive marijuana policies.

Change state laws to reduce or eliminate penalties for the medical and non-medical use of marijuana."

National Organization for the Reform of Marijuana Laws (NORML)
   https://norml.org/
Founded in 1970, the National Organization for the Reform of Marijuana Laws' mission is "to move public opinion sufficiently to legalize the responsible use of marijuana by adults, and to serve as an advocate for consumers to assure they have access to high quality marijuana that is safe, convenient and affordable." Their website contains extensive legal information about the drug, including state-by-state policy reports, news releases, a library, and information on campaigns and advocacy.

Medical Professionals

American Cannabis Nurses Association (ACNA)
   https://cannabisnurses.org/
ACNA is an organization for nurses and other medical providers who need information about medical cannabis. The group's mission is "to advance excellence in cannabis nursing practice through advocacy, collaboration, education, research and policy development." There are regional groups and conferences, and the website contains resources for patients and medical providers.

American Medical Marijuana Physicians Association (AMMPA)
   https://ammpa.net/
AMMPA is a membership-driven organization that educates physicians and other healthcare providers on cannabis as a medicine. The group holds an annual meeting and their website contains both legal and educational resources.

Society of Cannabis Clinicians (SCC)
   http://www.cannabisclinicians.org/
This organization is a "nonprofit educational and scientific society of qualified physicians and other professionals dedicated to the promotion, protection and support of cannabis for medical use." Based in California, SCC's website provides resources, a list of practitioners and information on continuing education for cannabis providers.

General Information on Medical Marijuana

Center for Medicinal Cannabis Research
https://www.cmcr.ucsd.edu/index.php
The website of the UC Center for Cannabis Research has a wealth of information on medical cannabis, including links to studies, investigators, news, and publications, as well as an FAQ section.

Healer
https://healer.com/
Founded by a doctor of osteopathy from Arizona, Healer provides cannabis education links, dosage programs for patients, and training for healthcare providers.

International Cannabinoid Research Society (ICRS)
http://icrs.co/
The ICRS is an organization dedicated to "research about cannabinoids in all fields." The website notes, "In addition to acting as a source for impartial information on cannabis and the cannabinoids, the main role of the ICRS is to provide an open forum for researchers to meet and discuss their research." While the site is primarily for member scientists, it does feature links to recently published studies.

Leafly: Cannabis 101
https://www.leafly.com/news/cannabis-101
Leafly is a commercial site with links to dispensaries, product reviews, and more. For those just starting to use marijuana, however, the "Cannabis 101" section offers basic information on buying cannabis, consumption methods, different strains, and laws.

Project CBD
https://www.projectcbd.org/
Project CBD is "a California-based nonprofit dedicated to promoting and publicizing research into the medical uses of cannabidiol (CBD) and other components of the cannabis plant." Their website is a compendium of news about cannabis from newspapers, journals, and online sources. There is also a beginner's guide to cannabis therapy that is especially helpful for new patients.

"O'Shaughnessy's"

https://beyondthc.com/

Started as a print journal of marijuana news and information, *O'Shaugh-nessy's* online contains the archives of the newspapers as well as a compendium of news and information about the plant.

State Medical Cannabis Laws as of December 2018[*]

*Information in this graph is adapted from National Conference of State Legislatures website, http://www.ncsl.org/research/health/state-medical-marijuana-laws.aspx.

State	Laws	Allows Dispensaries	Specifies Conditions	Recognizes Patients from Other States
ALASKA	Meas. 8 (1998) SB 94 (1999) Statute Title 17, Chapter 37	Yes	Yes	No
ARIZONA	Proposition 203 (2010)	Yes	Yes	Yes for AZ approved conditions. No for dispensary purchases
ARKANSAS	Issue 6 (2016) *Details pending*	Pending	Pending	Pending
CALIFORNIA	Proposition 215 (1996) SB 420 (2003)	Yes	No	No
COLORADO	Amendment 20 (2000)	Yes	Yes	No
CONNECTICUT	HB 5389 (2012)	Yes	Yes	Yes
DELAWARE	SB 17 (2011)	Yes	Yes	Yes, for DE approved conditions
DIST. OF COLUMBIA	Initiative 59 (1998) L18–0210 (2010)	Yes	Yes	Yes
FLORIDA	Amendment 2 (2016) *Details pending*	Pending	Pending	Pending

Hawaii	HB 862 (2000)	Yes	Yes	No
Illinois	HB 1 (2013)	Yes	Yes	No
Louisiana	SB 271 (2017) *Not yet in effect*	Yes	Yes	No
Maine	Question 2 (1999) LD 611 (2002) Question 5 (2009) LD 1811 (2010) LD 1296 (2011)	Yes	Yes	Yes, but not for dispensary purchases
Maryland	HB 702 (2003) SB 308 (2011) HB 180/SB 580 (2013) HB 1101-Chapter 403 (2013) SB 923 (2014)	Yes	Yes	No
Massachusetts	Question 3 (2012)	Yes	Yes	No
Michigan	Proposal 1 (2008)	Not in state law but localities may create ordinances to allow them	Yes	Yes, but not for dispensary purchases
Minnesota	SF 2471, Chapter 311 (2014)	Yes, limited liquid extract products only	Yes	No
Missouri	Amendment 2 (2018) *Details pending*	Pending	Yes	To be determined

State	Laws	Allows Dispensaries	Specifies Conditions	Recognizes Patients from Other States
MONTANA	Initiative 148 (2004) SB 423 (2011) Initiative 182 (2016)	No. New details pending	Yes	No. New details pending
NEVADA	Question 9 (2000)	Yes	Yes	Yes, if the other state's program is "substantially similar"
NEW HAMPSHIRE	HB 573 (2013)	Yes	Yes	Yes, with a note from home state but no dispensary purchases
NEW JERSEY	SB 119 (2009)	Yes	Yes	No
NEW MEXICO	SB 523 (2007)	Yes	Yes	No
NEW YORK	A6357 (2014)	Yes. Ingested doses may not contain more than 10 mg THC and product may not be combusted (smoked)	Yes	No
NORTH DAKOTA	Measure 5 (2016) Details pending	Yes	Yes	No
OHIO	HB 523 (2016) Not yet operational	Yes	Yes	Pending
OKLAHOMA	HB 788 (2018) Not yet operational	Pending	Pending	Pending

State	Legislation			
OREGON	Oregon Medical Marijuana Act (1998) SB 161 (2007)	Yes	Yes	No
PENNSYLVANIA	SB 3 (2016) *Not yet operational*	Yes	Yes	Pending
RHODE ISLAND	SB 791 (2007) SB 185 (2009)	Yes	Yes	Yes
UTAH	Proposition 2 (2018)	Yes	Yes	To be determined
VERMONT	SB 76 (2004) SB 7 (2007) SB 17 (2011) H.511 (2018)	Yes	Yes	No
WASHINGTON	Initiative 692 (1998) SB 5798 (2010) SB 5073 (2011)	Yes, as of 2014	Yes	No
WEST VIRGINIA	SB 386 (2017)	Yes. No whole flower for sale and cannot be smoked (but may be vaporized)	Yes	No

States with Limited Access Medical Cannabis Laws (CBD-only)

Alabama	South Carolina
Georgia	Tennessee
Iowa	Texas
Indiana	Virginia
Kentucky	Wisconsin
Mississippi	Wyoming
North Carolina	

States with Full Adult Access to Cannabis (Legal for Anyone 21+)

Alaska	Massachusetts
California	Michigan
Colorado	Nevada
District of Columbia	Oregon
Illinois	Vermont
Maine	Washington

Chapter Notes

Preface

1. While cannabis is the accepted medical term for the plant and drug, it has generated a variety of terms in English throughout history. Hemp, a common English term for cannabis, once referred to the plant in all of its forms but now generally refers to northern varieties grown for their fiber. Marijuana is probably the most universally recognized term for the plant and was a Spanish term popularized by prohibitionists in the U.S. during the 1930s in a racist attempt to associate the drug with Mexicans. Of course, there are also a variety of slang terms associated with cannabis, including weed, Mary Jane, reefer, pot, dope, and bud. While cannabis is the preferred term, especially in a medicinal sense, I will vary my terminology throughout this text for reasons of style.

Introduction

1. *Merriam-Webster OnLine,* s.v. "pioneer" (accessed September 17, 2016), www.merriam-webster.com/dictionary.

2. Ibid., "refugee."

3. "Colorado Gold Rush," *Colorado Encyclopedia*, https://coloradoencyclopedia.org/article/colorado-gold-rush.

4. Ibid.

5. Richard Gehling, "The Pike's Peak Gold Rush, 1858–1860," 1999, https://web.archive.org/web/20080628172253/http://www.geocities.com/Heartland/Falls/2000/index.html.

6. Ibid.

7. Ibid.

8. Nick Lindsey, "More Than 200,000 People Moved to Colorado Between 2013–2014," October 15, 2015, www.greenrushdaily.com/2015/10/15/200000-people-moved-to-colorado.

9. "According to a New Survey, 4 out of Every 5 People Move to Colorado for Marijuana," *Denver City Page*, January 3, 2016, www.imfromdenver.com/according-to-a-new-survey-4-out-of-every-5-people-move-to-colorado-for-marijuana.

10. "Medical Marijuana Access in the United States," Americans for Safe Access, 2017 Annual Report, www.safeaccessnow.org/.

11. Americans for Safe Access website.

12. Martin A. Lee, *Smoke Signals: A Social History of Marijuana: Medical, Recreational, and Scientific* (New York: Scribner, 2012), 3–4.

13. Ibid., 5–6.

14. Ibid., 5.

15. Ibid.

16. Ibid., 22–23.

17. Ibid., 24.

18. Ibid., 26.

19. David Newton, *Marijuana: A Reference Handbook* (ABC-CLIO, 2013), http://www.myilibrary.com?ID=45362, 37.

20. Christopher Ingraham, "The DEA Chief Called Medical Marijuana 'a Joke.' Now Patients Are Calling for His Resignation," *Washington Post*, November 10, 2015, https://www.washingtonpost.com/news/wonk/wp/2015/11/10/the-dea-chief-called-

medical-marijuana-a-joke-now-patients-are-calling-for-his-resignation/?utm_term=.1e40d63fbc94.

21. "Anslinger, Harry Jacob, and U.S. Drug Policy." *Encyclopedia of Drugs, Alcohol, and Addictive Behavior*, 2001, Encyclopedia.com, https://www.encyclopedia.com/education/encyclopedia-almanacs-transcripts-and-maps/anslinger-harry-jacob-and-us-drug-policy/.

22. Johann Hari, *Chasing the Scream: The First and Last Days of the War on Drugs* (New York: Bloomsbury, 2015), 11–13.

23. Cydney Adams, "The Man Behind the Marijuana Ban for All the Wrong Reasons," November 17, 2016, http://www.cbsnews.com/news/harry-anslinger-the-man-behind-the-marijuana-ban/.

24. Hari, *Chasing the Scream*, 14–15.

25. Ibid., 16.

26. Ibid., 17.

27. Lee, *Smoke Signals*, 54.

28. "Richard Nixon: Remarks About an Intensified Program for Drug Abuse Prevention and Control—June 17, 1971," The American Presidency Project, http://www.presidency.ucsb.edu/ws/?pid=3047.

29. Erik Sherman, "Nixon's Drug War, an Excuse to Lock Up Blacks and Protesters, Continues," *Forbes*, March 23, 2016, http://www.forbes.com/sites/eriksherman/2016/03/23/nixons-drug-war-an-excuse-to-lock-up-blacks-and-protesters-continues/#7e07c98a5099.

30. "A Brief History of the Drug War," Drug Policy Alliance, http://www.drugpolicy.org/facts/new-solutions-drug-policy/brief-history-drug-war-0.

31. Peter Wagner and Bernadette Rabuy, "Mass Incarceration: The Whole Pie, 2016," *Prison Policy Initiative*, March 14, 2016, https://www.prisonpolicy.org/reports/pie2016.html.

32. "Drug War Statistics," Drug Policy Alliance, http://www.drugpolicy.org/drug-war-statistics.

33. Tom Angell, "Marijuana Arrests Are Increasing Despite Legalization, New FBI Data Shows," *Forbes,* September 24, 2018, https://www.forbes.com/sites/tomangell/2018/09/24/marijuana-arrests-are-increasing-despite-legalization-new-fbi-data-shows/#1467de454c4b.

34. "Drug War Statistics," Drug Policy Alliance, http://www.drugpolicy.org/drug-war-statistics.

35. Michael Roberts, "Remembering Jack Splitt: MMJ Jack's Law Namesake Loses Fight for Life," *Westword*, August 26, 2016, http://www.westword.com/news/remembering-jack-splitt-mmj-jacks-law-namesake-loses-fight-for-life-7982321.

36. Colorado Department of Public Health and Environment. "Medical Marijuana Statistics and Data," https://www.colorado.gov/pacific/cdphe/medical-marijuana-statistics-and-data.

37. State of Colorado, "Department of Public Health and Environment," 2017, https://www.colorado.gov/pacific/cdphe/approved-medical-marijuana-research-grants.

38. Sonja Haug, "Migration Networks and Migration Decision Making," *Journal of Ethnic and Migration Studies* 34, no. 4 (May 2008): 585–605, https://doi.org/10.1080/13691830801961605.

Chapter 1

1. Crohn's and Colitis Foundation of America, http://www.crohnscolitisfoundation.org/what-are-crohns-and-colitis/what-is-crohns-disease/crohns-medication.html.

2. I will use the terms "western" and "conventional" medicine in this book when discussing allopathic medicine and the standard medical establishment in the U.S and Europe.

3. The bud or "flower" of the cannabis plant contains the highest concentrations of cannabinoids, including THC, responsible for marijuana's "high," and CBD, with various medicinal properties. In order to release the cannabinoids' properties, the bud must be heated (which is why it is often smoked) or captured in heated oil (cannabis is oil soluble) for edible products. Cannabinoids can also be extracted with alcohol or another solvent.

4. Epilepsy Foundation, 2016, www.epilepsy.com.

5. Saundra Young, "Marijuana Stops Child's Severe Seizures," *CNN,* August 7, 2013 (accessed October 4, 2016), http://www.cnn.com/2013/08/07/health/charlotte-child-medical-marijuana/index.html.

6. Ibid.

7. www.epilepsy.com.

8. Ibid.

9. Annette Ogbru, "Benzodiazepines," RXList, May 2, 2016, http://www.rxlist.com/benzodiazepines/drugs-condition.htm.

10. John P. Cunha, "Depakote ER Side Effects," RXList, September 23, 2016, http://www.rxlist.com/depakote-er-side-effects-drug-center.htm.

11. "What Is the Glasgow Coma Scale?" http://www.brainline.org/content/2010/10/what-is-the-glasgow-coma-scale.html.

12. www.epilepsy.com.

13. Zerrin Atakan, "Cannabis, a Complex Plant: Different Compounds and Different Effects on Individuals," *Therapeutic Advances in Psychopharmacology* 2, no. 6 (2012): 241–254, https://doi.org/10.1177/2045125312457586.

14. Vincenzo Di Marzo, "A Brief History of Cannabinoid and Endocannabinoid Pharmacology as Inspired by the Work of British Scientists," *Trends in Pharmacological Sciences* 27, no. 3 (March 2006): 134–40, doi:10.1016/j.tips.2006.01.010.

15. Ibid.

16. Ibid.

17. Ethan B. Russo, "Taming THC: Potential Cannabis Synergy and Phytocannabinoid-Terpenoid Entourage Effects." *British Journal of Pharmacology* 163, no. 7 (2011): 1344–1364, *PMC,* doi: 10.1111/j.1476-5381.2011.01238.x.

18. "Working to Reform Marijuana Laws," National Organization for the Reform of Marijuana Laws, http://norml.org/legal/medical-marijuana-2.

19. Sy Mukherjee, "This Company Made the First FDA Approved, Marijuana Based Drug. Here's What It Wants to Do Next," *Fortune,* June 27, 2018, http://fortune.com/2018/06/27/fda-marijuana-gw-pharma-epidiolex-whats-next/.

20. Andrew Pollack, "Marijuana-Based Drug Found to Reduce Epileptic Seizures," *New York Times,* March 15, 2016, https://www.nytimes.com/2016/03/15/business/marijuana-based-drug-found-to-reduce-epileptic-seizures.html?_r=0.

21. Ibid.

22. www.epilepsy.com

23. Mitchell, Thomas. "Medical Marijuana for Autism Law Approved on World Autism Day." *Westword,* April 2, 2019. https://www.westword.com/marijuana/colorado-celebrates-world-autism-day-by-legalizing-medical-marijuana-for-autism-11296161.

24. www.epilepsy.com.

25. Jeremy Kossen, "How Does Cannabis Consumption Affect Autism?" May 19, 2016, https://www.leafly.com/news/health/how-does-cannabis-consumption-affect-autism.

26. Evan Halper, "DEA Ends Its Monopoly on Marijuana Growing for Medical Research," *Los Angeles Times,* August 11, 2016, http://www.latimes.com/politics/la-na-marijuana-dea-20160811-snap-story.html.

Chapter 2

1. Epilepsy Foundation, www.epilepsy.com, 2016.

2. Rudy Mawer, "The Ketogenic Diet 101: A Beginner's Guide," *Healthline,* June 17, 2017, https://www.healthline.com/nutrition/ketogenic-diet-101.

3. Max Davidson, "New Jersey Gov. Agrees to Possible Changes to Medical Marijuana Law," April 6, 2014, http://www.thedailychronic.net/2014/30488/new-jersey-governor-agrees-to-possible-changes-to-medical-marijuana-law/.

4. http://www.cannabilityfoundation.org/.

5. Bente Birkeland, "Colorado Schools Have Been Slow to Allow Medical Marijuana, Lawmakers Want a Change," Aspen Public Radio, http://aspenpublicradio.org/post/colorado-schools-have-been-slow-allow-medical-marijuana-lawmakers-want-change#stream/0.

6. www.cannabilityfoundation.org.

7. Ibid.

8. Monte Whaley, "Colorado Districts Wrestle with New Law Allowing Students to Use Medical Marijuana at School," *Denver Post*, August 22, 2016, http://www.denverpost.com/2016/08/22/schools-medical-marijuana-jacks-law/.

9. Jen Christensen, "Groundbreaking Medical Marijuana Case Lets Little Girl Go Back to School," cnn.com, April 27, 2018, https://www.cnn.com/2018/01/22/health/medical-marijuana-school-illinois/index.html.

10. "Gov. Rauner Signs Bill Allowing Medical Marijuana for Students at Illinois Public Schools," *Chicago Tribune*, August 2, 2018, http://www.chicagotribune.com/news/local/breaking/ct-met-rauner-school-marijuana-20180802-story.html.

11. Jen Christensen and Dan Simon, "Girl Can Attend School with Her Cannabis-based Medicine, California Court Rules," cnn.com, September 25, 2018, https://www.cnn.com/2018/09/25/health/medical-marijuana-california-child-school-ruling/index.html.

12. Ryan Glasspiegel, "Medical Marijuana: Colorado Law Continues Implementation," *Huffington Post*, August 16, 2012, http://www.huffingtonpost.com/ryan-glasspiegel/medical-marijuana-colorado-denver_b_1602632.html.

13. "History of Colorado's Marijuana Laws," 2013, http://sensiblecolorado.org/history-of-co-medical-marijuana-laws/.

14. www.sensiblecolorado.org.

15. "Samantha Spady: Another College Alcohol Overdose Death," in *I Speak of Dreams*, http://lizditz.typepad.com/i_speak_of_dreams/2004/12/samantha_spady_.html.

16. Angie Wagner, "Night of Partying Proves Deadly for Popular Student," *Los Angeles Times*, November 28, 2004, http://articles.latimes.com/2004/nov/28/news/adna-drinkdeath28/2.

17. "Blood Alcohol Concentration and Calculator," *Aware Awake Alive*, http://awareawakealive.org/educate/blood-alcohol-content.

18. "Gordie's Story," Gordie Center, UVA, https://gordiecenter.studenthealth.virginia.edu/gordie/gordies-story.

19. Melia Robinson, "Here's How Much Marijuana It Would Take to Kill You," *Business Insider*, November 5, 2016, https://www.businessinsider.com/can-marijuana-kill-you-2016-11.

20. National Institute on Drug Abuse, "Drug Facts: Marijuana," revised June 2018, https://www.drugabuse.gov/publications/drugfacts/marijuana.

21. "Vital Signs: Alcohol Poisoning Deaths—United States, 2010–2012," *Morbidity and Mortality Weekly Report* 65, no. 53 (January 9, 2015): 1238–1242, https://www.cdc.gov/mmwr/preview/mmwrhtml/mm6353a2.htm?s_cid=mm6353a2_w.

22. National Institute on Drug Abuse, "Overdose Death Rates," revised August 2018, https://www.drugabuse.gov/related-topics/trends-statistics/overdose-death-rates.

23. Mason Tvert, interview with author, January 19, 2017.

24. William Breathes, "The History of Cannabis in Colorado … or How the State Went to Pot," *Westword*, November 1, 2012, http://www.westword.com/news/the-history-of-cannabis-in-coloradoor-how-the-state-went-to-pot-5118475.

25. *Colorado Amendment 64: Use and Regulation of Marijuana*, http://www.fcgov.com/mmj/pdf/amendment64.pdf.

26. "Fibromyalgia," Mayo Clinic, September 8, 2016, http://www.mayoclinic.org/diseases-conditions/fibromyalgia/basics/definition/con-20019243.

27. Colorado (State), Legislature, General Assembly, *Prevent Marijuana Diversion to Illegal Market* (HB17–1220, pre-amended), 2017 Regular Session, Colorado General Assembly, https://openstates.org/co/bills/2017A/HB17–1220/.

28. Stuart S. Taylor, "Marijuana Policy and Presidential Leadership: How to Avoid a Federal-State Train Wreck," Brookings, July 28, 2016, https://www.brookings.edu/research/marijuana-policy-and-presidential-leadership-how-to-avoid-a-federal-state-train-wreck/.

29. "USDOJ New Policy," October 19, 2009, http://medicalmarijuana.procon.org/sourcefiles/USDOJNewPolicy.pdf.

30. Tim Dickinson, "Obama's War on Pot," *Rolling Stone*, February 16, 2012, http://www.rollingstone.com/politics/news/obamas-war-on-pot-20120216.

31. "The Cole Memo: 8 Federal Guidelines on Marijuana Law Enforcement," *Cannabist*, http://www.thecannabist.co/2014/02/14/cole-memo-federal-law-enforcement-guidelines-on-marijuana-enforcement/4733/.

32. Taylor, "Marijuana Policy and Presidential Leadership."

33. Erik Eckholm, "Medical Marijuana Industry Is Unnerved by U.S. Crackdown," *New York Times*, November 23, 2011, http://www.nytimes.com/2011/11/24/us/medical-marijuana-target-of-us-prosecutors.html?mcubz=2.

34. ProCon, "Should Marijuana Be a Medical Option?" http://medicalmarijuana.procon.org/view.additional-resource.php?resourceID=000149.

35. Mike Riggs, "Obama's War on Pot," *The Nation*, June 29, 2015, https://www.thenation.com/article/obamas-war-pot/.

36. Dana Rohrabacher, "H.Amdt.748 to H.R.4660–113th Congress (2013–2014)," Congress.gov, May 30, 2014, https://www.congress.gov/amendment/113th-congress/house-amendment/748.

37. Ed Perlmutter, "Text—H.R.2652–113th Congress (2013–2014): Marijuana Businesses Access to Banking Act of 2013," Congress.gov, September 13, 2013, https://www.congress.gov/bill/113th-congress/house-bill/2652/text.

38. "BSA Expectations Regarding Marijuana-Related Businesses," FinCEN.gov, https://www.fincen.gov/resources/statutes-regulations/guidance/bsa-expectations-regarding-marijuana-related-businesses.

39. "Frequently Asked Questions: Marijuana and Banking," February 2014, https://www.aba.com/Tools/Comm-Tools/Documents/ABAMarijuanaAndBankingFAQFeb2014.pdf.

40. Thomas Mitchell, "Long Odds for Reintroduced Marijuana Banking Bill," *Westword*, April 2, 2016, http://www.westword.com/news/long-odds-for-reintroduced-marijuana-banking-bill-6674809.

Chapter 3

1. "Genetic and Rare Diseases Information Center," National Institutes of Health, 2017, https://rarediseases.info.nih.gov/diseases.

2. "Haleigh," Georgia's Hope, https://georgiashope.com/project/haleigh/.

3. "Working to Reform Marijuana Laws," National Organization for the Reform of Marijuana Laws, http://norml.org/legal/medical-marijuana-2.

4. Flowering Hope Foundation, http://www.floweringhope.co/.

5. Vanessa Waltz, "Interview: Jason Cranford on Haleigh's Hope, Colorado Medical Cannabis Laws, and the Realm of Caring Waiting List," *Ladybud*, April 2, 2014, http://www.ladybud.com/2014/04/02/interview-jason-cranford-on-haleighs-hope-colorado-medical-cannabis-laws-and-the-realm-of-caring-waiting-list/.

6. Richard Anderson, "Pharmaceutical Industry Gets High on Fat Profits," *BBC News*, November 6, 2014, http://www.bbc.com/news/business-28212223.

7. "CEO Reviled for Drug Price Hike Charged with Securities Fraud," CBS News, December 17, 2015, http://www.cbsnews.com/news/martin-shkreli-charged-with-securities-fraud/.

8. Jonathan D. Rockoff, "Mylan Faces Scrutiny Over Epipen Price Increases," *Wall Street Journal*, August 24, 2016, https://www.wsj.com/articles/mylan-faces-scrutiny-over-epipen-price-increases-1472074823.

9. Rick Mullin, "Cost to Develop New Pharmaceutical Drug Now Exceeds $2.5B," *Scientific American*, November 20, 2014, https://www.scientificamerican.com/article/cost-to-develop-new-pharmaceutical-drug-now-exceeds-2-5b/.

10. Anderson, "Pharmaceutical Industry Gets High on Fat Profits."

11. Ibid.

12. Colette DeJong, "Pharmaceutical

Industry–Sponsored Meals and Prescribing Patterns," *JAMA Internal Medicine*, August 1, 2016, http://jamanetwork.com/journals/jamainternalmedicine/article-abstract/2528290.

13. ProCon, "10 Pharmaceutical Drugs Based on Cannabis," http://medicalmarijuana.procon.org/view.resource.php?resourceID=000883.

14. GW Pharma, www.gwpharm.com, 2016.

15. S. Narang et al., "Efficacy of Dronabinol as an Adjuvant Treatment for Chronic Pain Patients on Opioid Therapy," *Journal of Pain: Official Journal of the American Pain Society* (March 2008), https://www.ncbi.nlm.nih.gov/pubmed/18088560.

16. Brian Montopoli, "Does the Pot Pill Work?" *CBS News*, August 3, 2009, http://www.cbsnews.com/news/does-the-pot-pill-work/.

17. Ibid.

18. Martin A. Lee, "Synthetic vs. Whole Plant CBD," in *Medical Marijuana*, https://www.projectcbd.org/article/synthetic-vs-whole-plant-cbd.

19. www.mpp.org

20. "Schizencephaly," Brainfacts.org, http://www.brainfacts.org/diseases-disorders/diseases-a-to-z-from-ninds/schizencephaly/.

Chapter 4

1. Bailey Rahn, "What Is THCA and What Are the Benefits of This Cannabinoid?" *Leafly*, March 17, 2015, https://www.leafly.com/news/cannabis-101/what-is-thca-and-what-are-the-benefits-of-this-cannabinoid.

2. Zillow, Inc., "Colorado Home Prices and Home Values," Zillow, https://www.zillow.com/co/home-values/.

3. Amelia Josephson, "The Cost of Living in Colorado," *SmartAsset*, August 15, 2016, https://smartasset.com/mortgage/the-cost-of-living-in-colorado.

4. Ibid.

5. "Refugee Admissions," U.S. Department of State, https://www.state.gov/j/prm/ra/.

6. Carly Willis, "Kansas Man Arrested After Growing Cannabis to Control Seizures," *KSNT News*, April 20, 2017, http://ksnt.com/2017/04/20/kansas-man-arrested-after-growing-cannabis-to-control-seizures/.

7. Saundra Young, "3-Year-Old Is Focus of Medical Marijuana Battle," CNN, January 15, 2014, http://www.cnn.com/2014/01/15/health/cannabis-landon-riddle/index.html.

8. Ibid.

9. Jessica Firger, "Cancer and Kids: Is Marijuana the Answer?" *Newsweek*, July 18, 2017, http://www.newsweek.com/2017/07/28/medical-marijuana-pediatric-cancer-637676.html.

10. Utah legalized medical marijuana shortly before this book went to press. It's to be hoped the Riddles will be able to return to Utah to visit without fear of legal repercussions in the near future.

11. Lisa Rough, "Can You Legally Transport Cannabis Across State Lines?" Leafly.com, June 23, 2017, https://www.leafly.com/news/cannabis-101/can-you-transport-cannabis-between-two-legal-states.

12. Jens Manuel Krogstad and Jynnah Radford, "Key Facts About Refugees to the U.S.," Pew Research Center, January 30, 2017, http://www.pewresearch.org/fact-tank/2017/01/30/key-facts-about-refugees-to-the-u-s/.

13. Megan Barber, "Refugees in American Cities: 5 Key Things to Know," *Curbed*, January 30, 2017, https://www.curbed.com/2017/1/30/14440160/refugees-united-states-cities.

14. Larisa Epatko, "Syrian Refugees Find a Safe Haven in Amish Country," PBS, http://www.pbs.org/newshour/updates/syrian-refugees-find-a-safe-haven-in-amish-country/.

15. Carlos Illescas, "Aurora Reaching Out to Refugee Community," *Denver Post*, May 21, 2016, http://www.denverpost.com/2013/12/21/aurora-reaching-out-to-refugee-community/.

16. Immigrant and Refugee Commission—City of Aurora, https://www.auroragov.org/city_hall/boards___commissions/immigrant_and_refugee_commission.

17. "Type I Glycogen Storage Disease," American Liver Foundation, http://www.liverfoundation.org/abouttheliver/info/gsdi/.

18. Ibid.

19. Maia Szalavitz, "Marijuana: The Next Diabetes Drug?" *Time,* May 21, 2013, http://healthland.time.com/2013/05/21/marijuana-the-next-diabetes-drug/.

Chapter 5

1. "Would You Risk Going to Jail to Ease Your Child's Suffering?" *Next,* October 23, 2015, http://www.nowtolove.co.nz/news/real-life/love-and-the-drug-6953.

2. Laura McQuillan, "Kiwis Are Literally Dying to Use Medicinal Cannabis. Is a Change to the System Bold Enough?" stuff.co.nz, June 2, 2017, http://www.stuff.co.nz/national/93284426/kiwis-are-literally-dying-to-use-medicinal-cannabis-is-a-change-to-the-system-bold-enough.

3. Ibid.

4. "Peter Dunne Says Medical Cannabis in Tragic Alex Renton Case Was Worthwhile," stuff.co.nz, July 2, 2015, http://www.stuff.co.nz/national/health/69888664/nelson-teenager-alex-renton-dies-despite-treatment-with-medical-cannabis.

5. "Alex Renton's Mother Hits Back at Cannabis Report," Radio New Zealand, January 18, 2016, http://www.radionz.co.nz/news/national/294312/mother-hits-back-at-cannabis-report.

6. Ibid.

7. "Rose Renton Petition for Medical Cannabis," *NORML New Zealand,* March 22, 2016, https://norml.org.nz/2016/sign-the-rose-renton-petition-for-medicinal-cannabis/.

8. Mei Heron, "Alex Renton's Mum Presents Reform Petition to Parliament," Radio New Zealand, October 13, 2016, http://www.radionz.co.nz/news/national/315470/alex-renton's-mum-presents-reform-petition-to-parliament.

9. Isaac Davison, "Restrictions on Medical Cannabis to be Removed," *New Zealand Herald,* June 2, 2017, http://www.nzherald.co.nz/nz/news/article.cfm?c_id=1&objectid=11868146.

10. Sam Levin, "Expots: Medical Marijuana Draws Parents to U.S. for Their Children's Treatments," *The Guardian,* May 9, 2016, https://www.theguardian.com/society/2016/may/09/medical-marijuana-families-move-to-colorado-epilepsy.

11. "Legality of Cannabis by Country," Wikipedia, April 16, 2017, https://en.wikipedia.org/wiki/Legality_of_cannabis_by_country.

12. Christopher Moraff, "The UN's Prohibitionism Impedes Drug Policy Reform," *Al Jazeera America,* http://america.aljazeera.com/opinions/2015/3/the-uns-prohibitionist-stance-impedes-drug-policy-reform.html.

13. United Nations Office on Drugs and Crime, "The 1912 Hague International Opium Convention," https://www.unodc.org/unodc/en/frontpage/the-1912-hague-international-opium-convention.html.

14. Ibid.

15. Martin Booth, *Cannabis: A History* (New York: Thomas Dunne Books/St. Martin's, 2004), 139.

16. Schaefer Library of Drug Policy, *Cannabis in Context, History, Laws, and International Treaties,* http://druglibrary.net/schaffer/Library/studies/aus/can_ch3.htm.

17. United Nations Single Convention on Narcotic Drugs, as Amended by the 1972 Protocol Amending the Single Convention on Narcotic Drugs, 1961, UNTS volume 976, p. 105, New York, https://www.incb.org/incb/en/narcotic-drugs/1961_Convention.html.

18. Moraff, "The UN's Prohibitionism Impedes Drug Policy Reform."

19. "Richard Nixon: Remarks About an Intensified Program for Drug Abuse Prevention and Control—June 17, 1971," The American Presidency Project, http://www.presidency.ucsb.edu/ws/?pid=3047.

20. Moraff, "The UN's Prohibitionism Impedes Drug Policy Reform."

21. Scott Gacek, "WHO Takes First Steps to Reclassify Marijuana Under Inter-

national Law," *Medical Jane,* January 1, 2017, https://www.medicaljane.com/2017/01/01/who-takes-first-steps-to-reclassify-medical-cannabis-under-international-law/.

22. Isabel Kershner, "Israel, a Medical Marijuana Pioneer, Is Eager to Capitalize," *New York Times,* December 17, 2016, https://www.nytimes.com/2016/12/17/world/middleeast/israel-a-medical-marijuana-pioneer-is-eager-to-capitalize.html?mcubz=2.

23. Yardena Schwartz, "The Holy Land of Medical Marijuana," USnews.com, April 11, 2017, https://www.usnews.com/news/best-countries/articles/2017-04-11/israel-is-a-global-leader-in-marijuana-research.

24. Kershner, "Israel, a Medical Marijuana Pioneer."

25. Karin Kloosterman, "Dr. 'Cannabis': Alan Shackelford Puts Medicine into Marijuana, in Israel," *Green Prophet,* January 20, 2015, https://www.greenprophet.com/2015/01/dr-cannabis-alan-shackelford-puts-medicine-into-cannabis-in-israel/.

26. "OWC Pharmaceutical Research Corp Release Company Issues Annual Letter to Shareholders," http://www.biospace.com/News/owc-pharmaceutical-research-corp-release-company/444409.

27. Gardiner Harris, "Researchers Find Study of Medical Marijuana Discouraged," *New York Times,* January 18, 2010, http://www.nytimes.com/2010/01/19/health/policy/19marijuana.html?mcubz=2.

28. Kloosterman, "Dr. 'Cannabis.'"

29. William Breathes, "Marijuana: Colorado Doc Alan Shackelford Conducting Cannabis Research in Israel," *Westword,* February 21, 2017, http://www.westword.com/news/marijuana-colorado-doc-alan-shackelford-conducting-cannabis-research-in-israel-6282409.

30. *Atlas Obscura,* "University of Mississippi Marijuana Research Project," http://www.atlasobscura.com/places/university-of-mississippi-marijuana-research-project.

31. Tamir Gedo, "Why Israel Leads the U.S. in Medical Cannabis Research," *Jerusalem Post* | JPost.com, March 16, 2017, http://www.jpost.com/Opinion/Why-Israel-leads-the-U.S.-in-medical-cannabis-research-484416.

32. Caleb Hellerman, "Scientists Say the Government's Only Pot Farm Has Moldy Samples," PBS, http://www.pbs.org/newshour/updates/scientists-say-governments-pot-farm-moldy-samples-no-guidelines/.

33. Ibid.

34. Maayan Lubell and Lianne Back, "Israel Looks to Leverage Tech in $50 Billion Medical Marijuana Market," Reuters, March 23, 2017, http://www.reuters.com/article/us-israel-cannabis-idUSKBN16U1PZ.

35. Ibid.

36. Gedo, "Why Israel Leads the U.S. in Medical Cannabis Research."

37. Craig A. Press et al., "Parental Reporting of Response to Oral Cannabis Extracts for Treatment of Refractory Epilepsy," *Epilepsy and Behavior* 45 (2015): 49–52, doi:10.1016/j.yebeh.2015.02.043.

38. Lauren Treat et al., "Duration of Use of Oral Cannabis Extract in a Cohort of Pediatric Epilepsy Patients," *Epilepsia* 58, no. 1 (2016): 123–27, doi:10.1111/epi.13617.

39. "Marijuana Research with Human Subjects," U.S. Food and Drug Administration Home Page, https://www.fda.gov/newsevents/publichealthfocus/ucm421173.htm.

40. "The Drug Development Process—Step 3: Clinical Research," U.S. Food and Drug Administration Home Page (accessed June 25, 2017), https://www.fda.gov/ForPatients/Approvals/Drugs/ucm405622.htm.

41. David Noonan, "Scientists Want the Smoke to Clear on Medical Marijuana Research," *Scientific American,* https://www.scientificamerican.com/article/scientists-want-the-smoke-to-clear-on-medical-marijuana-research/.

42. Ibid.

43. Ibid.

44. "DEA Ends Its Monopoly on Marijuana Growing for Medical Research," *Los Angeles Times,* http://www.latimes.com/politics/la-na-marijuana-dea-20160811-snap-story.html.

45. DEA/Drug Scheduling (accessed June 25, 2017), https://www.dea.gov/drug info/ds.shtml.

46. "Health Effects of Marijuana and Cannabis-Derived Products Presented in New Report," National Academies, http://www8.nationalacademies.org/onpinews/newsitem.aspx?RecordID=24625&_ga=1.172863584.235057739.1484262362.

47. Ibid.

48. Edward J. Hoffenberg et al., "Cannabis and Pediatric Inflammatory Bowel Disease," *Journal of Pediatric Gastroenterology and Nutrition* 64, no. 2 (2017): 265–71, doi:10.1097/mpg.0000000000001393.

49. Ibid.

50. Ibid.

Chapter 6

1. "Cumulative Concussions," Defense and Veterans Brain Injury Center, April 27, 2017, http://dvbic.dcoe.mil/audience/medical-providers.

2. Ibid.

3. Michael S. Jaffee, "Traumatic Brain Injury and the Military Health System," in *Systems Engineering to Improve Traumatic Brain Injury Care in the Military Health System: Workshop Summary,* Washington, D.C.: National Academies Press, 2009, https://www.ncbi.nlm.nih.gov/books/NBK214914/.

4. "NIH Fact Sheets—Post-Traumatic Stress Disorder (PTSD)," National Institutes of Health, U.S. Department of Health and Human Services, https://report.nih.gov/NIHfactsheets/ViewFactSheet.aspx?csid=58.

5. Ibid.

6. Ibid.

7. Ibid.

8. Anil Nischal et al., "Suicide and Antidepressants: What Current Evidence Indicates," *Mens Sana Monographs* 10, no. 1 (January–December 2012): 33–44, https://www.ncbi.nlm.nih.gov/pmc/articles/PMC3353604/.

9. Weed for Warriors Project, http://www.wfwproject.org/.

10. Chris Adams, "Millions Went to War in Iraq, Afghanistan, Leaving Many with Lifelong Scars," Mcclatchydc, http://www.mcclatchydc.com/news/nation-world/national/article24746680.html.

11. Ibid.

12. Weed for Warriors Project, http://www.wfwproject.org/.

13. Dave Philipps, "Suicide Rate Among Veterans Has Risen Sharply Since 2001," *New York Times*, July 7, 2016, https://www.nytimes.com/2016/07/08/us/suicide-rate-among-veterans-has-risen-sharply-since-2001.html.

14. "New VA Study Finds 20 Veterans Commit Suicide Each Day," *Military Times*, http://www.militarytimes.com/story/veterans/2016/07/07/va-suicide-20-daily-research/86788332/.

15. Phillips, "Suicide Rate Among Veterans Has Risen."

16. "DoD Worldwide Numbers for TBI," DVBIC, http://dvbic.dcoe.mil/dod-worldwide-numbers-tbi.

17. U.S. Department of Veterans Affairs, "How Common Is PTSD?" PTSD: National Center for PTSD, July 5, 2007, https://www.ptsd.va.gov/public/ptsd-overview/basics/how-common-is-ptsd.asp.

18. "New VA Study Finds 20 Veterans Commit Suicide Each Day, " *Military Times*, http://www.militarytimes.com/story/veterans/2016/07/07/va-suicide-20-daily-research/86788332/.

19. "Fort Hood Shooter Nidal Hasan Appears in Court Long After Death Sentence," *The Guardian*, January 29, 2015, https://www.theguardian.com/us-news/2015/jan/29/fort-hood-shooter-nidal-hasan-death-sentence-review.

20. Joe Davidson, "Will VA Chief Be Voice of Reason on Climate Change and Medical Marijuana in Trump Administration?" *Washington Post*, June 5, 2017, https://www.washingtonpost.com/news/powerpost/wp/2017/06/05/will-va-chief-be-voice-of-reason-on-climate-change-and-medical-marijuana-in-trump-administration/?hpid=hp_hp-cards_hp-card-fedgov%3Ahomepage%2Fcard&utm_term=.aca71f3b791b.

21. Ibid.

22. Ibid.

23. Joe Celli and Lou Plenzler, "What Wounded Veterans Need: Medical Marijuana," *Defense One*, May 26, 2017, http://www.defenseone.com/ideas/2017/05/what-wounded-veterans-need-medical-marijuana/138204/.

24. "Marijuana for Symptoms of PTSD in U.S. Veterans," MAPS, http://www.maps.org/research/mmj/marijuana-us.

25. Ibid.

26. Ibid.

27. Evan Halper, "Pot Researcher Abruptly Fired by University of Arizona," *Los Angeles Times*, July 1, 2014, http://www.latimes.com/nation/la-na-pot-researcher-fired-20140701-story.html.

28. "Marijuana for Symptoms of PTSD in U.S. Veterans," MAPS, http://www.maps.org/research/mmj/marijuana-us.

29. Perry Stein, "Veterans Drop Hundreds of Empty Pill Bottles in Front of the White House," *Washington Post*, November 11, 2015, https://www.washingtonpost.com/news/local/wp/2015/11/11/veterans-drop-hundreds-of-empty-pill-bottles-in-front-of-the-white-house/?utm_term=.f86ca9ca51d4.

30. Grow for Vets, https://growforvets.org/.

31. Veterans Cannabis Project, http://www.vetscp.org/#.

32. Colorado Department of Public Health and Environment, "Qualifying Medical Conditions Medical Marijuana Registry," https://www.colorado.gov/pacific/cdphe/qualifying-medical-conditions-medical-marijuana-registry.

33. Michael Roberts, "Inside Medical Marijuana Lawsuit Filed Against Colorado by Vets with PTSD," *Westword*, April 3, 2017, http://www.westword.com/news/inside-medical-marijuana-lawsuit-filed-against-colorado-by-vets-with-ptsd-7728656.

34. Ibid.

35. Ibid.

36. Thomas Mitchell, "Colorado Board of Health Rejects PTSD as MMJ Condition," *Westword*, April 2, 2016, http://www.westword.com/news/colorado-board-of-health-rejects-ptsd-as-mmj-condition-6915169.

37. Nick Schou, "PTSD-Stricken Marine Vet Faces Five Years in Oklahoma Prison for Growing Six Marijuana Plants," *OC Weekly*, March 8, 2017, http://www.ocweekly.com/news/ptsd-stricken-marine-vet-faces-five-years-in-oklahoma-prison-for-growing-six-marijuana-plants-7493535.

38. Amy Dawn Bourlon-Hiltebran, "Veteran Faces Life for Cannabis, Murderer Does Not," *MassRoots*, May 18, 2017, https://www.massroots.com/news/kristoffer-lewandowski-trial-oklahoma.

39. "USMC Veteran Facing Life in Prison Over 1 Oz. of Cannabis to Treat His PTSD," *Activist Post*, May 25, 2017, http://www.activistpost.com/2017/05/usmc-veteran-facing-life-prison-1-oz-cannabis-treat-ptsd.html.

40. "Domestic Disturbance Turns into Pot Bust," KSWO.com, June 2, 2014, http://www.kswo.com/story/25674226/domestic-disturbance-turns-into-pot-bust.

41. "Weed Warrior Kris Lewandowski No Longer Faces Life in Prison," *GFarma News*, June 8, 2017, http://gfarma.news/entertainment-news/weed-warrior-kris-lewandowski-no-longer-faces-life-prison/.

Conclusion

1. Mark Minton, "Banda Pleads Not Guilty; Medical Cannabis Experts Testify," *Garden City Telegram*, April 7, 2017, http://www.gctelegram.com/62e6748c-d9bd-5cfd-b900-c1516afebccf.html.

2. Brigid Schulte, "Mom Who Uses Medical Marijuana Faces Up to 30 Years in Prison," *Washington Post*, June 8, 2015, https://www.washingtonpost.com/news/local/wp/2015/06/08/mom-who-uses-medical-marijuana-faces-up-to-30-years-in-prison/?utm_term=.b4fdf8f44e3f.

3. Ibid.

4. Shona Banda, Interview by Ben Swann, *Ben Swann Radio Show*, YouTube, May 22, 2014, audio, 1:19:30, https://www.youtube.com/watch?v=sdJ1ScVUGm0.

5. C.J. Janovy, "Garden City 'Pot Mom' Pleads No Contest in Exchange for Probation," kcur.org, August 11, 2017, http://kcur.org/post/garden-city-pot-mom-pleads-no-contest-exchange-probation#stream/0.

6. Phillip Smith, "Mother Who Used Medical Cannabis to Treat Deadly Disease Had Her Son Taken Away, Faces 28 Years in Prison," *Alternet*, http://www.alternet.org/drugs/shona-banda-medical-marijuana-legal-nightmare-continues.

7. Ibid.

8. Minton, "Banda Pleads Not Guilty."

9. Janovy, "Garden City 'Pot Mom' Pleads No Contest."

10. Mark Minton, "Banda Sentenced to 12 Months Probation," *Garden City Telegram*, October 13, 2017, http://www.gctelegram.com/news/20171013/banda-sentenced-to-12-months-probation.

11. Josiah Hesse, "U.S. Veteran's Children Taken Away Over His Use of Medical Marijuana," *The Guardian,* February 1, 2016 (accessed January 29, 2017), https://www.theguardian.com/society/2016/feb/01/medical-marijuana-use-colorado-kansas-veteran-custody-battle?utm_source=esp&utm_medium=Email&utm_campaign=GU+Today+USA+-+Version+CB+header&utm_term=154188&subid=17486699&CMP=ema_565b.

12. Ibid.

13. Ibid.

14. Bill Draper et al., "Raymond, Amelia Schwab Had Numerous Legal Issues Before Kids Taken Away," WIBW, Topeka, Kansas, March 31, 2016, http://www.wibw.com/content/news/Raymond-Amelia-Schwab-had-numerous-run-ins-with-the-law-before-kids-taken-away-374202781.html.

15. Ibid.

16. Hesse, "U.S. Veteran's Children Taken Away."

17. Ibid.

18. Ibid.

19. "Court Papers Shine Light on Schwab Case," KSN-TV. April 11, 2016, http://ksn.com/2016/04/08/court-papers-shine-light-on-schwab-case/.

20. Melissa Brunner, "Schwabs Say Court Is Allowing Children to Return Home," wibw.com, November 20, 2017, https://www.wibw.com/content/news/Schwabs-say-Court-is-allowing-children-to-return-home-458952683.html.

21. Hesse, "U.S. Veteran's Children Taken Away."

22. Caroline Preston, "Parents Face Child Abuse Investigations Over Pot Use," *Al Jazeera America*, http://america.aljazeera.com/articles/2015/9/7/parents-face-child-abuse-investigations-over-marijuana-use.html.

23. "Parental Drug Use as Child Abuse," National Institutes of Health, U.S. Department of Health and Human Services, https://www.childwelfare.gov/pubPDFs/drugexposed.pdf.

24. Family Law and Cannabis Alliance, http://flcalliance.org/.

25. Preston, "Parents Face Child Abuse Investigations Over Pot Use."

26. Timothy Williams, "Marijuana Arrests Outnumber Those for Violent Crimes, Study Finds," *New York Times*, October 12, 2016, https://www.nytimes.com/2016/10/13/us/marijuana-arrests.html?mcubz=2.

27. Simon Thompson, "97% of Texas Marijuana Convictions Are for Possession," KRWG, http://krwg.org/post/97-texas-marijuana-convictions-are-possession.

28. Ibid.

29. Jesse Wegman, Opinion: "The Injustice of Marijuana Arrests," *New York Times*, July 28, 2014, https://www.nytimes.com/2014/07/29/opinion/high-time-the-injustice-of-marijuana-arrests.html?mcubz=2.

30. Tom Angell, "Marijuana Arrests Are Increasing Despite Legalization, New FBI Data Shows," *Forbes*, September 24, 2018, https://www.forbes.com/sites/tomangell/2018/09/24/marijuana-arrests-are-increasing-despite-legalization-new-fbi-data-shows/#1467de454c4b.

31. Drug Policy Alliance, "Drug War Statistics," http://www.drugpolicy.org/issues/drug-war-statistics.

32. ACLU, "Study Documents Extreme Racial Disparity in Arrests for Low-Level Offenses," December 21, 2015, https://www.aclu.org/news/study-documents-extreme-racial-disparity-arrests-low-level-offenses.

33. Benjamin Mueller, "Using Data to Make Sense of a Racial Disparity in NYC Marijuana Arrests," *New York Times*, May

13, 2018, https://www.nytimes.com/2018/05/13/insider/data-marijuana-arrests-racial-disparity.html.

34. Benjamin Mueller, Robert Gebeloff and Sahil Chinoy, "Surest Way to Face Marijuana Charges in New York: Be Black or Hispanic," *New York Times*, May 13, 2018, https://www.nytimes.com/2018/05/13/nyregion/marijuana-arrests-nyc-race.html?action=click&module=Related Coverage&pgtype=Article&region=Footer.

35. Preston, "Parents Face Child Abuse Investigations Over Pot Use."

36. Ibid.

37. Gloria Van Rees, "Woman with Terminal Cancer Jailed Over Medication in Her System," KAKE.com, May 3, 2017, http://www.kake.com/story/35335390/woman-with-terminal-cancer-jailed-over-medication-in-her-system.

38. Carly Willis, "Kansas Man Arrested After Growing Cannabis to Control Seizures," *KSNT News*, April 20, 2017, http://ksnt.com/2017/04/20/kansas-man-arrested-after-growing-cannabis-to-control-seizures/.

39. Safer Lock, "The Secret Danger for Parents Who Smoke Medical Marijuana," December 9, 2015, https://saferlockrx.com/the-secret-danger-for-parents-who-smoke-medical-marijuana/.

Epilogue

1. Jamie Corroon and Rod Kight, "The Evolving Regulatory Status of Cannabidiol," *Project CBD Newsletter*, November 26, 2018, https://www.projectcbd.org/about/legal-issues/evolving-regulatory-status-cannabidiol.

2. Aaron Cadena, "Is CBD Legal? The Legal Status of CBD in 2018," medium.com, January 22, 2018, https://medium.com/cbd-origin/is-cbd-legal-legal-status-of-cbd-2018-d1b4a0ed42df.

3. John Hudak, "The Farm Bill, Hemp Legalization and the Status of CBD: An Explainer," Brookings, December 14, 2018, https://www.brookings.edu/blog/fixgov/2018/12/14/the-farm-bill-hemp-and-cbd-explainer/.

4. Ibid.

5. Ibid.

6. Ibid.

7. Sy Mukherjee, "This Company Made the First FDA Approved, Marijuana Based Drug. Here's What It Wants to Do Next," *Fortune*, June 27, 2018, http://fortune.com/2018/06/27/fda-marijuana-gw-pharma-epidiolex-whats-next/.

8. Elaine Watson, "What Is the Regulatory Status of CBD in Food and Beverage Products?" *Food navigator-usa.com*, October 10, 2018, https://www.foodnavigator-usa.com/Article/2018/10/11/SPECIAL-FEATURE-What-is-the-regulatory-status-of-CBD-in-food-and-beverage-products.

9. Christopher Ingraham, "Jeff Sessions Personally Asked Congress to Let Him Prosecute Medical-Marijuana Providers," *Washington Post*, June 13, 2017, https://www.washingtonpost.com/news/wonk/wp/2017/06/13/jeff-sessions-personally-asked-congress-to-let-him-prosecute-medical-marijuana-providers/?utm_term=.eab89766b083.

10. Sadie Gurman, "Huff, Puff, Pass? AG's Pot Fury Not Echoed by Task Force," APNews, August 5, 2017, https://apnews.com/ad37624fcb8e485a8d57a013d48a227c.

11. Matt Laslo, "How the Pot Movement Changed in 2018," *Rolling Stone*, December 24, 2018, https://www.rollingstone.com/culture/culture-features/marijuana-weed-2018-changed-pot-772473/.

12. Danny Reed, "What Does Trump AG Pick William Barr Mean for the Cannabis Industry?" *MG*, December 13, 2018, https://mgretailer.com/cannabis-news/what-does-trump-ag-pick-william-barr-mean-for-cannabis-industry/.

13. Polly Washburn, "Public Support for Medical and Recreational Marijuana Legalization Hits All-Time High," *Cannabist*, August 8, 2017, http://www.thecannabist.co/2017/08/08/marijuana-legalization-opinion-poll-americans/85562/.

14. Ibid.

15. Alex Pasquariello, "Cannabis Industry Org Forms to 'Be Ready' for National Legalization," *Cannabist*, http://www.thecannabist.co/2017/06/16/national-association-of-cannabis-businesses-marijuana-industry/81746/.

16. Ibid.

17. Debra Borchardt, "Marijuana Sales Totaled $6.7 Billion in 2016," *Forbes*, January 3, 2017, https://www.forbes.com/sites/debraborchardt/2017/01/03/marijuana-sales-totaled-6-7-billion-in-2016/#6635194075e3.

18. Ibid.

19. Alicia Wallace, "America's Marijuana Industry Headed for $24 Billion by 2025," *Cannabist,* February 22, 2017, http://www.thecannabist.co/2017/02/22/report-united-states-marijuana-sales-projections-2025/74059/.

20. Alicia Wallace, " Medical Marijuana Could Poach More Than $4B from Pharma Sales Annually," *Cannabist*, May 24, 2017, http://www.thecannabist.co/2017/05/24/medical-marijuana-pharmaceutical-sales-impact/80045/.

21. Tom Schuba, "Cannabis 101: A Guide to Medical Marijuana in Illinois," *Chicago Sun Times*, September 5, 2018, https://chicago.suntimes.com/cannabis/illinois-medical-marijuana-law-dispensaries-cannabis/.

22. Ibid.

References

"According to a New Survey, 4 out of Every 5 People Move to Colorado for Marijuana." *Denver City Page,* January 3, 2016. http://www.imfromdenver.com/according-to-a-new-survey-4-out-of-every-5-people-move-to-colorado-for-marijuana/.

ACLU. "Study Documents Extreme Racial Disparity in Arrests for Low-Level Offenses." December 21, 2015. https://www.aclu.org/news/study-documents-extreme-racial-disparity-arrests-low-level-offenses.

Adams, Chris. "Millions Went to War in Iraq, Afghanistan, Leaving Many with Lifelong Scars." *Mcclatchydc.* http://www.mcclatchydc.com/news/nation-world/national/article24746680.html.

Adams, Cydney. "The Man Behind the Marijuana Ban for All the Wrong Reasons." *CBS News.* November 17, 2016. http://www.cbsnews.com/news/harry-anslinger-the-man-behind-the-marijuana-ban/.

Adams, Mike. "California Rep. Rohrabacher Introduces Bill to End Federal Marijuana Prohibition in Legal States." *Merry Jane,* February 10, 2017. https://www.merryjane.com/news/federal-bill-designed-to-end-marijuana-prohibition-in-2017.

_____. "Congress Members to VA: Let Veterans Smoke Marijuana." *High Times,* January 29, 2016. http://hightimes.com/news/politics/congress-members-to-va-let-veterans-smoke-marijuana/.

Agorist, Matt. "USMC Veteran Facing Life in Prison Over 1 Oz. of Cannabis to Treat His PTSD." *Activist Post,* May 25, 2017. http://www.activistpost.com/2017/05/usmc-veteran-facing-life-prison-1-oz-cannabis-treat-ptsd.html.

Allsop, Josh. "GW Pharmaceuticals's Cannabidiol Epilepsy Drug Ready for NDA Filing." *Proactive Investors,* August 9, 2016. http://www.proactiveinvestors.com/companies/news/129158/gw-pharmaceuticals-s-cannabidiol-epilepsy-drug-ready-for-nda-filing-129158.html.

Alsever, Jennifer. "Is Pot Losing Its Buzz in Colorado?" *Fortune,* June 19, 2016. http://fortune.com/pot-marijuana-colorado/?iid=sr-link1.

American Liver Foundation. "Type I Glycogen Storage Disease." http://www.liverfoundation.org/abouttheliver/info/gsdi/.

"American Medical Refugees Foundation." *Dope,* March 15, 2017. http://www.dopemagazine.com/tag/american-medical-refugees-foundation/.

The American Presidency Project. "Richard Nixon: Remarks About an Intensified Program for Drug Abuse Prevention and Control—June 17, 1971." http://www.presidency.ucsb.edu/ws/?pid=3047.

Americans for Safe Access. "House and Senate CARERS Act Petition." http://www.safeaccessnow.org/senate_carers_act_petition.

Americans for Safe Access website. March 2016. http://www.safeaccessnow.org/.

"Amy Sue Root." 2016. https://www.caringbridge.org/visit/amysueroot.ca

Andavolu, Krishna (host). *Weediquette.* Episode 3, "Marijuana Minors." VICE Video. https://video.vice.com/en_us/video/stoned-kids/5609651ec70bd226563be353.

Anderson, Richard. "Pharmaceutical Industry Gets High on Fat Profits." *BBC News.* November 6, 2014. http://www.bbc.com/news/business-28212223.

Angell, Tom. "Marijuana Arrests Are Increasing Despite Legalization, New FBI Data Shows." *Forbes,* September 24, 2018. https://www.forbes.com/sites/tomangell/2018/09/24/marijuana-arrests-are-increasing-despite-legalization-new-fbi-data-shows/#1467de454c4b.

"Anslinger, Harry Jacob, and U.S. Drug Policy." *Encyclopedia of Drugs, Alcohol, and Addictive Behavior,* 2001. Encyclopedia.com. https://www.encyclopedia.com/education/encyclopedias-almanacs-transcripts-and-maps/anslinger-harry-jacob-and-us-drug-policy.

Antonacci, Karen. "For Colorado Veterans, Marijuana a Controversial Treatment." *Longmont Times-Call,* November 5, 2016. http://www.timescall.com/longmont-local-news/ci_30542597/colorado-veterans-marijuana-controversial-treatment.

Atakan, Zerrin. "Cannabis, a Complex Plant: Different Compounds and Different Effects on Individuals." *Therapeutic Advances in Psychopharmacology* 2, no. 6 (2012): 241–254. https://doi.org/10.1177/2045125312457586.

Atlas Obscura. "University of Mississippi Marijuana Research Project." http://www.atlasobscura.com/places/university-of-mississippi-marijuana-research-project.

"Average Colorado Springs Home Price Hits Record High in January." *Colorado Springs Gazette,* February 6, 2017. http://gazette.com/average-colorado-springs-home-price-hits-record-high-in-january/article/1596158.

Baca, Ricardo. "Year in Weed: The Five Most Important Medical Marijuana Research Studies of 2016." *Cannabist,* December 30, 2016. http://www.thecannabist.co/2016/12/30/marijuana-research-of-2016/69971/.

Banda, Shona. Interview by Ben Swann. *Ben Swann Radio Show,* YouTube, May 22, 2014. Audio, 1:19:30. https://www.youtube.com/watch?v=sdJ1ScVUGm0.

Barber, Megan. "Refugees in American Cities: 5 Key Things to Know." *Curbed,* January 30, 2017. https://www.curbed.com/2017/1/30/14440160/refugees-united-states-cities.

Barcott, Bruce. *Weed the People: The Future of Legal Marijuana in America.* New York: Time, 2015.

"The Best American Cities for Refugees Share These Key Qualities." *Quartz,* September 19, 2016. https://qz.com/783276/the-best-american-cities-for-refugees-share-these-key-qualities/.

Billing, Geoff. Interview with the author, March 3, 2017.

Biospace. "OWC Pharmaceutical Research Corp Release Company Issues Annual Letter to Shareholders." http://www.biospace.com/News/owc-pharmaceutical-research-corp-release-company/444409.

Birkeland, Bente. "Colorado Schools Have Been Slow to Allow Medical Marijuana; Lawmakers Want a Change." Aspen Public Radio. April 13, 2016. http://aspenpublicradio.org/post/colorado-schools-have-been-slow-allow-medical-marijuana-lawmakers-want-change#stream/0.

Blissken, Snake. "Not So Fast: Veteran with PTSD Fighting Harsh Sentence for Growing His Own Medicine." *High Times,* January 9, 2017. http://hightimes.com/culture/not-so-fast-veteran-with-ptsd-fighting-harsh-sentence-for-growing-his-own-medicine/.

"Blood Alcohol Concentration and Calculator." *Aware Awake Alive.* http://awareawakealive.org/educate/blood-alcohol-content.

Bolognini, D., and R.A. Ross. "Medical Cannabis vs. Synthetic Cannabinoids: What Does the Future Hold?" *Clinical Pharmacology and Therapeutics* 97, no. 6 (May 9, 2015): 568–70. https://doi.org/10.1002/cpt.107.

Booth, Martin. *Cannabis: A History.* New York: Thomas Dunne Books/St. Martin's Press, 2004.

Borchardt, Debra. "Desperate Parents of Autistic Children Trying Cannabis Despite Lack of Studies." *Forbes*, June 10, 2015. http://www.forbes.com/sites/debraborchardt/2015/06/10/desperate-parents-of-autistic-children-trying-cannabis-despite-lack-of-studies/#3f0ca7812c94.

_____. "Marijuana Sales Totaled $6.7 Billion in 2016." *Forbes*, January 3, 2017. https://www.forbes.com/sites/debraborchardt/2017/01/03/marijuana-sales-totaled-6-7-billion-in-2016/#6635194075e3.

Bostwick, J. Michael. "Blurred Boundaries: The Therapeutics and Politics of Medical Marijuana." *Mayo Clinic Proceedings* 87, no. 2 (February 2012): 172–86. https://doi.org/10.1016/j.mayocp.2011.10.003.

Bourlon-Hiltebran, Amy Dawn. Interview with the author, September 2, 2015 and May 9, 2017.

_____. "Veteran Faces Life for Cannabis, Murderer Does Not." *MassRoots*, May 18, 2017. https://www.massroots.com/news/kristoffer-lewandowski-trial-oklahoma.

"Brain Malformations." *MedlinePlus*. https://medlineplus.gov/brainmalformations.html.

Brainfacts.org. "Schizencephaly." http://www.brainfacts.org/diseases-disorders/diseases-a-to-z-from-ninds/schizencephaly/.

Brainline. "What Is the Glasgow Coma Scale?" http://www.brainline.org/content/2010/10/what-is-the-glasgow-coma-scale.html.

Breathes, William. "The History of Cannabis in Colorado … or How the State Went to Pot." *Westword*. http://www.westword.com/news/the-history-of-cannabis-in-color adoor-how-the-state-went-to-pot-5118475.

_____. "Marijuana: Colorado Doc Alan Shackelford Conducting Cannabis Research in Israel." *Westword*, February 21, 2017. http://www.westword.com/news/marijuana-colorado-doc-alan-shackelford-conducting-cannabis-research-in-israel-6282409.

Brunner, Melissa. "Schwabs Say Court Is Allowing Children to Return Home." wibw.com. November 20, 2017. https://www.wibw.com/content/news/Schwabs-say-Court-is-allowing-children-to-return-home-458952683.html.

"BSA Expectations Regarding Marijuana-Related Businesses." FinCEN.gov. https://www.fincen.gov/resources/statutes-regulations/guidance/bsa-expectations-regarding-marijuana-related-businesses.

Bunker, Barbara. Interview with the author, May 9, 2016.

_____. "Sleepwalker." Sweet Super Nova (blog). May 8, 2016. http://sweetsupernova.weebly.com/blog.

Cadena, Aaron. "Is CBD Legal?: The Legal Status of CBD in 2018." medium.com. January 22, 2018. https://medium.com/cbd-origin/is-cbd-legal-legal-status-of-cbd-2018-d1b4a0ed42df.

"Can Marijuana Heal a Wounded Warrior?" *CBS News*. June 25, 2014. http://www.cbsnews.com/news/marijuana-debate-veterans-using-pot-to-treat-ptsd-and-war-wounds/.

CannAbility Foundation. "Consider Her Canna Able: Stacey Linn and the CannAbility Foundation." July 2015. http://www.cannabilityfoundation.org/.

"Cannabis and Autism—A Partnership for the Better?" Updated 2010. http://www.cannabissearch.com/medical_benefits/autism/.

"Cannabis in Context, History, Laws, and International Treaties." Schaefer Library of Drug Policy. http://druglibrary.net/schaffer/Library/studies/aus/can_ch3.htm.

Cannabis Patients Alliance. "Rx MaryJane." https://cannabispatientsalliance.org/author/rxmaryjane/.

CannabisNursesMagazine.com. March 10, 2017. https://cannabisnursesmagazine.com/.

Cannatol. Welcome Page. http://www.cannatol.com/cannatol-rx.

Caring Bridge. "Olivia Domer." 2016. https://www.caringbridge.org/visit/oliviadomer/journal/view/id/52898c29a589b40175964c02.

Castle, Shay. "Boulder County's Cannabis Innovators Have Big Plans for 2016." *Boulder Daily Camera*, December 12, 2015. http://www.dailycamera.com/boulder-business/ci_29236521/boulder-countys-cannabis-innovators-have-big-plans-2016.

_____. "What Bubble? Boulder County Ranked as Most Stable Housing Market in U.S." *Boulder Daily Camera*, July 6, 2016. http://www.dailycamera.com/boulder-business/ci_30098975/what-bubble-boulder-county-ranked-most-stable-housing.

Caulkins, Jonathan P., and Angela Hawken. *Marijuana Legalization: What Everyone Needs to Know*. Oxford: Oxford University Press, USA, 2012.

Celli, Joe, and Lou Plenzler. "What Wounded Veterans Need: Medical Marijuana." *Defense One*. May 26, 2017. http://www.defenseone.com/ideas/2017/05/what-wounded-veterans-need-medical-marijuana/138204/.

Centers for Disease Control and Prevention. "Traumatic Brain Injury and Concussion." April 27, 2017. https://www.cdc.gov/traumaticbraininjury/get_the_facts.html.

"CEO Reviled for Drug Price Hike Charged with Securities Fraud." *CBS News*. December 17, 2015. http://www.cbsnews.com/news/martin-shkreli-charged-with-securities-fraud/.

Childears, Don A. "Banking Marijuana Requires 'Act of Congress.'" http://c.ymcdn.com/sites/www.coloradobankers.org/resource/resmgr/imported/MJ%20Summary%20Reasons%2020020714.pdf.

Children's Hospital Colorado. "Medical Marijuana for Tumors." https://www.childrenscolorado.org/pediatric-innovation/research/cancer-research/medical-marijuana-for-central-nervous-system-tumors-research/.

_____. "Pediatric Research Areas." https://www.childrenscolorado.org/pediatric-innovation/research/.

Chilkoti, Avantika. "States Keep Saying Yes to Marijuana Use. Now Comes the Federal No." *New York Times*, July 15, 2017. https://www.nytimes.com/2017/07/15/us/politics/marijuana-laws-state-federal.html?mcubz=2.

Christensen, Jen. "Groundbreaking Medical Marijuana Case Lets Little Girl Go Back to School." CNN.com, April 27, 2018. https://www.cnn.com/2018/01/22/health/medical-marijuana-school-illinois/index.html.

Christensen, Jen, and Dan Simon. "Girl Can Attend School With Her Cannabis-Based Medicine, California Court Rules." CNN.com, September 25, 2018. https://www.cnn.com/2018/09/25/health/medical-marijuana-california-child-school-ruling/index.html.

Ciaramella, C.J. "The Heartbreaking Plight of Colorado's 'Marijuana Refugees.'" VICE.com, April 23, 2015. https://www.vice.com/en_us/article/jmaew3/the-heartbreaking-plight-of-colorados-marijuana-refugees-423.

Cloos, Kassondra. "Colorado Springs Student Suspended for Bringing Medical Marijuana to School." *Gazette*, May 14, 2015. http://gazette.com/colorado-springs-student-suspended-for-bringing-medical-marijuana-to-school/article/1551881.

Coleman, Shawn. Interview with the author, June 9, 2017.

Collective Evolution. "What Happened When They Treated Autistic Children with Medical Cannabis." February 17, 2015. http://www.collective-evolution.com/2015/02/17/what-happened-when-they-treated-autistic-children-with-medical-cannabis/.

Colorado Amendment 64: Use and Regulation of Marijuana. http://www.fcgov.com/mmj/pdf/amendment64.pdf

Colorado Department of Public Health and Environment. "Approved Medical Marijuana Research Grants." https://www.colorado.gov/pacific/cdphe/approved-medical-marijuana-research-grants.

_____. "Marijuana Fact Sheets in Multiple Languages." https://www.colorado.gov/pacific/cdphe/marijuana-fact-sheets.

_____. "Medical Marijuana Statistics and Data." https://www.colorado.gov/pacific/cdphe/medical-marijuana-statistics-and-data.

_____. "Marijuana Research." https://www.colorado.gov/pacific/cdphe/marijuana-research.

_____. "Marijuana Use." https://www.colorado.gov/pacific/cdphe/marijuanause.

_____. "Qualifying Medical Conditions Medical Marijuana Registry." https://www.colorado.gov/pacific/cdphe/qualifying-medical-conditions-medical-marijuana-registry.

Colorado Encyclopedia. "Colorado Gold Rush." https://coloradoencyclopedia.org/article/colorado-gold-rush.

"The Colorado Gold Rush." *Western Mining History.* http://www.westernmininghistory.com/articles/11/page1.

"Colorado Medical Marijuana Patients on Edge over Potential Trump Crackdown." *Colorado Springs Gazette*, May 17, 2017. http://gazette.com/colorado-medical-marijuana-patients-on-edge-over-potential-trump-crackdown/article/1603340.

"Colorado Medical Pot Law Poised to Add PTSD as Qualifier." *Denver Post*, October 2, 2016. http://www.denverpost.com/2016/09/21/colorado-medical-pot-law-ptsd/.

"Colorado Medical Use of Marijuana, Initiative 20 (2000)." Ballotpedia. https://ballotpedia.org/Colorado_Medical_Use_of_Marijuana,_Initiative_20_(2000).

"Colorado State Cost of Living." *Sperling's Best Places.* http://www.bestplaces.net/cost_of_living/state/colorado.

Colorado (State) Legislature. General Assembly. Allow Medical Marijuana Use for Stress Disorders (SB17–017). 2017 Regular Session. Colorado General Assembly. https://leg.colorado.gov/bills/sb17–017.

_____. General Assembly. Prevent Marijuana Diversion to Illegal Market (HB17–1220, preamended). 2017 Regular Session. Colorado General Assembly. https://openstates.org/co/bills/2017A/HB17–1220/.

Colorado State University Pueblo. "Institute of Cannabis Research." https://www.csupueblo.edu/institute-of-cannabis-research/.

Common Sense for Drug Policy. "CBS Questions Marinol's Efficacy." http://www.csdp.org/news/news/medmar_marinolCBS_080409.htm.

Cornerstone Collective. "How Far We've Come: A History of Endocannabinoid Research." December 1, 2014. http://cornerstonecollective.com/how-far-weve-come-a-history-of-endocannabinoid-research/.

"Correction: Medical Marijuana-Custody Story." *AP News*, March 31, 2016. https://apnews.com/850b4e93fb2b407c821cd3e01f8d7c66/man-says-marijuana-not-legal-scrapes-led-kids-removal.

Corroon, Jamie, and Rod Kight. "The Evolving Regulatory Status of Cannabidiol." *Project CBD Newsletter*, November 26, 2018. https://www.projectcbd.org/about/legal-issues/evolving-regulatory-status-cannabidiol.

"Couple Fighting for Custody of 5 Kids Gets Help from Medical Pot Advocates." *CBS Denver*, June 12, 2017. http://denver.cbslocal.com/2017/06/12/medical-marijuana-ptsd-child-custody/.

"Court Papers Shine Light on Schwab Case." KSN-TV. April 11, 2016. http://ksn.com/2016/04/08/court-papers-shine-light-on-schwab-case/.

Cranford, Jason. Interview with the author, September 3, 2015.

Crohn's and Colitis Foundation of America. "Crohn's Disease Medication Options." http://www.crohnscolitisfoundation.org/what-are-crohns-and-colitis/what-is-crohns-disease/crohns-medication.html.

Cunha, John P. "Depakote ER Side Effects." RXList. September 23, 2016. http://www.rxlist.com/depakote-er-side-effects-drug-center.htm.

Curthoys, Kathleen. "Clinical Trial Using Marijuana to Treat PTSD in Veterans Gets Underway." *Army Times*, February 7, 2017. https://www.armytimes.com/articles/clinical-trial-using-marijuana-to-treat-ptsd-in-veterans-gets-underway.

Davidson, Joe. "Will VA Chief Be Voice of Reason on Climate Change and Medical Marijuana in Trump Administration?" *Washington Post*, June 5, 2017. https://www.washingtonpost.com/news/powerpost/wp/2017/06/05/will-va-chief-be-voice-of-reason-on-climate-change-and-medical-marijuana-in-trump-administration/?hpid=hp_hp-cards_hp-card-fedgov%3Ahomepage%2Fcard&utm_term=.aca71f3b791b.

Davidson, Max. "New Jersey Gov. Agrees to Possible Changes to Medical Marijuana Law." *Daily Chronic*, April 6, 2014. http://www.thedailychronic.net/2014/30488/new-jersey-governor-agrees-to-possible-changes-to-medical-marijuana-law/.

Davison, Isaac. "Restrictions on Medical Cannabis to Be Removed." *New Zealand Herald*, June 2, 2017. http://www.nzherald.co.nz/nz/news/article.cfm?c_id=1&objectid=11868146.

DEA. "Drug Scheduling." https://www.dea.gov/druginfo/ds.shtml.

Defense and Veterans Brain Injury Center. "Cumulative Concussions." April 27, 2017. http://dvbic.dcoe.mil/audience/medical-providers.

_____. "DoD Worldwide Numbers for TBI." http://dvbic.dcoe.mil/dod-worldwide-numbers-tbi.

_____. "TBI and the Military." January 23, 2017. http://dvbic.dcoe.mil/tbi-military.

DeJong, Colette. "Pharmaceutical Industry—Sponsored Meals and Prescribing Patterns." *JAMA Internal Medicine*, August 1, 2016. http://jamanetwork.com/journals/jamainternalmedicine/article-abstract/2528290.

Democracy Now. "Marijuana Refugees: Virginia Family Moves to Colorado to Treat Epileptic Child with Cannabis Oil." January 10, 2017. https://www.democracynow.org/2014/5/9/marijuana_refugees_virginia_family_moves_to

Denver Post. "The Cole Memo: 8 Federal Guidelines on Marijuana Law Enforcement." *Cannabist*, February 14, 2014. http://www.thecannabist.co/2014/02/14/cole-memo-federal-law-enforcement-guidelines-on-marijuana-enforcement/4733/.

Di Marzo, Vincenzo. "A Brief History of Cannabinoid and Endocannabinoid Pharmacology as Inspired by the Work of British Scientists." *Trends in Pharmacological Sciences* 27, no. 3 (March 2006): 134–40. https://doi.org/10.1016/j.tips.2006.01.010.

Dickinson, Tim. "Obama's War on Pot." *Rolling Stone*, February 16, 2012. http://www.rollingstone.com/politics/news/obamas-war-on-pot-20120216.

Domer, Cara. Interview with the author, September 4, 2015.

Domer, Olivia. Interview with the author, February 10, 2016

"Domestic Disturbance Turns into Pot Bust." *ABC News*. June 2, 2014. http://www.kswo.com/story/25674226/domestic-disturbance-turns-into-pot-bust.

Draper, Bill, Melissa Hellman, and Nick Viviani. "Raymond, Amelia Schwab Had Numerous Legal Issues Before Kids Taken Away." WIBW | Topeka, Kansas. March 31, 2016. http://www.wibw.com/content/news/Raymond-Amelia-Schwab-had-numerous-run-ins-with-the-law-before-kids-taken-away-374202781.html.

Drug Policy Alliance. "A Brief History of the Drug War." http://www.drugpolicy.org/facts/new-solutions-drug-policy/brief-history-drug-war-0.

_____. "As a Medical Marijuana Patient, Where Can I Use or Get Access to Medicine While Traveling Abroad?" http://www.drugpolicy.org/blog/medical-marijuana-patient-where-can-i-use-or-get-access-medicine-while-traveling-abroad.

_____. "Drug War Statistics." http://www.drugpolicy.org/drug-war-statistics

_____. "Louisianan Given 13-Year Prison Sentence for Possession of Two Marijuana

Cigarettes." April 16, 2014. http://www.drugpolicy.org/news/2014/04/louisianan-given-13-year-prison-sentence-possession-two-marijuana-cigarettes.

Drugs.com. "Seroquel: Drug Uses, Dosage and Side Effects." https://www.drugs.com/seroquel.html.

Drury, Adam. "Governor of Colorado Rejects Medical Marijuana for Autism Treatment." *High Times*, June 6, 2018. https://hightimes.com/news/governor-colorado-rejects-medical-marijuana-autism-treatment/.

Eckholm, Erik. "Medical Marijuana Industry Is Unnerved by U.S. Crackdown." *New York Times*, November 23, 2011. http://www.nytimes.com/2011/11/24/us/medical-marijuana-target-of-us-prosecutors.html?mcubz=2.

El-Sohly, Mahmoud, ed. *Marijuana and the Cannabinoids.* Totowa, NJ: Humana, 2007.

Epatko, Larisa. "Syrian Refugees Find a Safe Haven in Amish Country." PBS. December 31, 2015. http://www.pbs.org/newshour/updates/syrian-refugees-find-a-safe-haven-in-amish-country/.

Epilepsy Foundation. http://www.epilepsy.com/.

Face of Cannabis. *NOVA.* August 11, 2014. https://faceofcannabis.wordpress.com/2014/08/11/nova/ (accessed January 29, 2017).

Family Law and Cannabis Alliance. http://flcalliance.org/.

Fine, Doug. *Too High to Fail: Cannabis and the New Green Economic Revolution.* New York: Gotham, 2012.

Firger, Jessica. "Cancer and Kids: Is Marijuana the Answer?" *Newsweek,* July 18, 2017. http://www.newsweek.com/2017/07/28/medical-marijuana-pediatric-cancer-637676.html.

Flowering Hope. "Power of Hope: Haleigh." http://www.floweringhope.co/power-of-hope-haleigh.html (accessed April 3, 2017).

Flowering Hope Foundation. http://www.floweringhope.co/.

Foreman, Nick. Interview with the author, June 2, 2017.

"Fort Hood Shooter Nidal Hasan Appears in Court Long After Death Sentence." *The Guardian,* January 29, 2015. https://www.theguardian.com/us-news/2015/jan/29/fort-hood-shooter-nidal-hasan-death-sentence-review.

Fowlie, Chris. Interview with the author, March 15, 2017.

"Frequently Asked Questions: Marijuana and Banking." February 2014. https://www.aba.com/Tools/Comm-Tools/Documents/ABAMarijuanaAndBankingFA.

"From 2500 Seizures a Month Without Cannabis to Zero with Cannabis." Episode 65. *Cannabis Health Radio.* January 25, 2017. https://cannabishealthradio.com/2017/01/episode-65-from-2500-seizures-a-month-without-cannabis-to-zero-with-cannabis/.

Frontline. "How Independent Is the FDA?" PBS. November 13, 2003. http://www.pbs.org/wgbh/pages/frontline/shows/prescription/hazard/independent.html.

_____. "Marijuana Timeline." PBS. http://www.pbs.org/wgbh/pages/frontline/shows/dope/etc/cron.html.

Gacek, Scott. "WHO Takes First Steps to Reclassify Marijuana Under International Law." *Medical Jane,* January 1, 2017. https://www.medicaljane.com/2017/01/01/who-takes-first-steps-to-reclassify-medical-cannabis-under-international-law/.

Gedo, Tamir. "Why Israel Leads the US in Medical Cannabis Research." *Jerusalem Post,* March 16, 2017. http://www.jpost.com/Opinion/Why-Israel-leads-the-US-in-medical-cannabis-research-484416.

Gehling, Richard. "The Pike's Peak Gold Rush, 1858–1860." 1999. https://web.archive.org/web/20080628172253/http://www.geocities.com/Heartland/Falls/2000/index.html.

Georgia's Hope. "Haleigh." https://georgiashope.com/project/haleigh/.

Ginn, Lori. Interview with the author, August 3, 2016.

Glasspiegel, Ryan. "Medical Marijuana: Colorado Law Continues Implementation." *Huffington Post*, August 16, 2012. http://www.huffingtonpost.com/ryan-glasspiegel/medical-marijuana-colorado-denver_b_1602632.html.

Glover, Lacie. "How Doctors Make Money from Drug Companies." *US News and World Report*, July 15, 2015. http://health.usnews.com/health-news/patient-advice/articles/2015/07/15/how-doctors-make-money-from-drug-companies.

Goldman, Marina, Jesse J. Suh, Kevin G. Lynch, Regina Szucs, Jennifer Ross, Hu Xie, Charles P. O'Brien, and David W. Oslin. "Identifying Risk Factors for Marijuana Use Among Veterans Affairs Patients." *Journal of Addiction Medicine* 4, no. 1 (March 2010): 45–49. https://doi.org/10.1097/adm.0b013e3181b18782.

"Gov. Rauner Signs Bill Allowing Medical Marijuana for Students at Illinois Public Schools." *Chicago Tribune*, August 2, 2018. http://www.chicagotribune.com/news/local/breaking/ct-met-rauner-school-marijuana-20180802-story.html.

Grant, Kelli B. "Marijuana Refugees Face Real Estate Challenges." CNBC. February 4, 2014. https://www.cnbc.com/2014/02/04/marijuana-refugees-face-real-estate-challenges.html.

Gray, Haley. "Colorado Adds PTSD as Qualifying Condition for Medical Marijuana." *5280*. April 28, 2017. http://www.5280.com/2017/04/colorado-adds-first-psychological-condition-for-medical-cannabis/.

Green, Johnny. "How Many Different Cannabinoids Are There in Marijuana?" *The Weed Blog*. May 31, 2015. https://www.theweedblog.com/how-many-different-cannabinoids-are-there-in-marijuana/.

Greene, Charlo. "Marijuana News, Product Reviews and Information." http://charlogreene.com.

Grinspoon, Lester, and James B Bakalar. *Marihuana, the Forbidden Medicine*. New Haven: Yale University Press, 1997.

Grotenhermen, Franjo, and Ethan B. Russo. *Cannabis and Cannabinoids: Pharmacology, Toxicology, and Therapeutic Potential*. New York: Haworth Integrative Healing, 2002.

Grow for Vets. https://growforvets.org/.

"Guidance 2014 G001—Financial Crimes Enforcement Network." February 14, 2014. https://www.fincen.gov/sites/default/files/shared/FIN-2014-G001.pdf.

Guo, Jeff. "Where Refugees Go in America." *Washington Post*, September 11, 2015. https://www.washingtonpost.com/news/wonk/wp/2015/09/11/where-refugees-go-in-america/?utm_term=.3f9bab506c83.

Gupta, Sanjay. *Weed—Dr. Sanjay Gupta Reports*. Aired August 11, 2013, on CNN. https://www.youtube.com/watch?v=Z3IMfIQ_K6U.

Gurman, Sadie. "Huff, Puff, Pass? AG's Pot Fury Not Echoed by Task Force." *AP News*. August 5, 2017. https://apnews.com/ad37624fcb8e485a8d57a013d48a227c.

GW Pharma. https://www.gwpharm.com/.

Haleigh's Hope™. https://haleighshope.com/.

Hall, Rocky. Interview with the author, May 4, 2017.

Halper, Evan. "DEA Ends Its Monopoly on Marijuana Growing for Medical Research." *Los Angeles Times*, August 11, 2016. http://www.latimes.com/politics/la-na-marijuana-dea-20160811-snap-story.html.

_____. "Pot Researcher Abruptly Fired by University of Arizona." *Los Angeles Times*, July 1, 2014. http://www.latimes.com/nation/la-na-pot-researcher-fired-20140701-story.html.

Hari, Johann. *Chasing the Scream: The First and Last Days of the War on Drugs*. New York: Bloomsbury, 2015.

Harris, Gardiner. "Researchers Find Study of Medical Marijuana Discouraged." *New York Times*, January 18, 2010. http://www.nytimes.com/2010/01/19/health/policy/19marijuana.html?mcubz=2.

Haug, Sonja. "Migration Networks and Migration Decision Making." *Journal of Ethnic and Migration Studies* 34, no. 4 (May 2008): 585–605. https://doi.org/10.1080/1369 1830801961605.

Hellerman, Caleb. "Scientists Say the Government's Only Pot Farm Has Moldy Samples." PBS. March 8, 2017. Accehttp://www.pbs.org/newshour/updates/scientists-say-governments-pot-farm-moldy-samples-no-guidelines/.

Helmuth, Josh. "Marijuana Refugees: Kansas Family Plans Move to Colorado for Medical Cannabis to Save Daughter." Kshb.com. February 20, 2016. http://www.kshb.com/news/local-news/marijuana-refugees-kansas-family-considers-moving-to-colorado-to-find-a-cannabis-cure-their-child.

Hernandez, Erica. "San Antonio 'Medical Refugees' Relocate for Legalized Marijuana to Aid Son." KSAT. February 22, 2017. http://www.ksat.com/health/medical-marijuana/medical-refugees-medical-marijuana-autism-epilepsy.

Heron, Mei. "Alex Renton's Mum Presents Reform Petition to Parliament." Radio New Zealand. October 13, 2016. http://www.radionz.co.nz/news/national/315470/alex-renton's-mum-presents-reform-petition-to-parliament.

Hesse, Josiah. "US Veteran's Children Taken Away Over His Use of Medical Marijuana." *The Guardian*, February 1, 2016. https://www.theguardian.com/society/2016/feb/01/medical-marijuana-use-colorado-kansas-veteran-custody-battle?utm_source=esp&utm_medium=Email&utm_campaign=GU+Today+USA+-+Version+CB+header&utm_term=154188&subid=17486699&CMP=ema_565b.

High Times, February 19, 2016. "10 Top-Rated States for Medical Marijuana." http://hightimes.com/culture/10-top-rated-states-for-medical-marijuana/.

History Colorado. "The Mining Industry in Colorado." March 23, 2011. http://www.historycolorado.org/content/mining-industry-colorado.

Hoffenberg, Ed. Interview with the author, May 19, 2017.

Hoffenberg, Edward J., Heike Newman, Colm Collins, Sally Tarbell, and Kristina Leinwand. "Cannabis and Pediatric Inflammatory Bowel Disease." *Journal of Pediatric Gastroenterology and Nutrition* 64, no. 2 (2017): 265–71. https://doi.org/10.1097/mpg.0000000000001393.

Honan, Megan, and Chris Nazarenus. "Jaxs' Policy." *Medical Marijuana 411*, May 13, 2016. https://medicalmarijuana411.com/jaxs-policy-colorado-approves-medical-marijuana-use/.

Hudak, John. "The Farm Bill, Hemp Legalization and the Status of CBD: An Explainer." Brookings. December 14, 2018. https://www.brookings.edu/blog/fixgov/2018/12/14/the-farm-bill-hemp-and-cbd-explainer/.

_____. "Why the CARERS Act Is So Significant for Marijuana Policy Reform." Brookings. July 29, 2016. https://www.brookings.edu/blog/fixgov/2016/04/13/why-the-carers-act-is-so-significant-for-marijuana-policy-reform/.

Huff, Ethan A. "Marijuana Cannabinoids Found to Help Combat Autism." *Natural News*, October 6, 2012. http://www.naturalnews.com/037445_marijuana_cannabinoids_autism.html.

I Speak of Dreams. "Samantha Spady: Another College Alcohol Overdose Death." http://lizditz.typepad.com/i_speak_of_dreams/2004/12/samantha_spady_.html.

Illescas, Carlos. "Aurora Reaching Out to Refugee Community." *Denver Post*, May 21, 2016. http://www.denverpost.com/2013/12/21/aurora-reaching-out-to-refugee-community/.

Immigrant and Refugee Commission—City of Aurora. https://www.auroragov.org/city_hall/boards___commissions/immigrant_and_refugee_commission.

"Influence of the United States on UN Drug Policy." *Mexico Voices*. http://mexicovoices.blogspot.com/p/inflluence-of-us-on-un-drug-policy.html.

Ingold, John. "CBD in Colorado: Seeking a Marijuana Miracle." *Denver Post*, 2014. http://extras.denverpost.com/stateofhope/.

Ingraham, Christopher. "The DEA Chief Called Medical Marijuana 'a Joke.' Now Patients Are Calling for His Resignation." *Washington Post*, November 10, 2015. https://www.washingtonpost.com/news/wonk/wp/2015/11/10/the-dea-chief-called-medical-marijuana-a-joke-now-patients-are-calling-for-his-resignation/?utm_term=.1e40d63fbc94.

_____. "Every Minute, Someone Gets Arrested for Marijuana Possession in the U.S." *Washington Post*, September 28, 2015. https://www.washingtonpost.com/news/wonk/wp/2015/09/28/every-minute-someone-gets-arrested-for-marijuana-possession-in-the-u-s/?utm_term=.c22a956628a2.

_____. "Jeff Sessions Personally Asked Congress to Let Him Prosecute Medical-Marijuana Providers." *Washington Post*, June 13, 2017. https://www.washingtonpost.com/news/wonk/wp/2017/06/13/jeff-sessions-personally-asked-congress-to-let-him-prosecute-medical-marijuana-providers/?utm_term=.eab89766b083.

_____. "Marijuana Has Truly Gone Mainstream, Survey Finds." *Washington Post*, April 19, 2017. http://www.denverpost.com/2017/04/19/marijuana-mainstream-study-finds/?preview_id=2621718.

_____. "Police Arrest More People for Marijuana Use Than for All Violent Crimes Combined." *Washington Post*, October 12, 2016. https://www.washingtonpost.com/news/wonk/wp/2016/10/12/police-arrest-more-people-for-marijuana-use-than-for-all-violent-crimes-combined/?utm_term=.087ce048ce79.

International Narcotics Control Board. Single Convention on Narcotic Drugs, 1961. https://www.incb.org/incb/en/narcotic-drugs/1961_Convention.html.

Iversen, Leslie L. *The Science of Marijuana*. New York: Oxford University Press, 2000.

"'Jack's Law': Medical Marijuana in Schools Bill Signed by Governor." CBS. June 7, 2016. http://denver.cbslocal.com/2016/06/07/jacks-law-medical-marijuana-in-schools-bill-signed-by-governor/.

Jaeger, Kyle. "What I Learned from Medical Marijuana Refugee Families." *attn:*, April 20, 2016. http://www.attn.com/stories/7132/medical-marijuana-refugee-families-in-colorado.

Jaffee, Michael S. "Traumatic Brain Injury and the Military Health System." In *Systems Engineering to Improve Traumatic Brain Injury Care in the Military Health System: Workshop Summary*. Washington, D.C.: National Academies Press, 2009. https://www.ncbi.nlm.nih.gov/books/NBK214914/.

Janovy, C.J. "Garden City 'Pot Mom' Pleads No Contest in Exchange for Probation." kcur.org. August 11, 2017. http://kcur.org/post/garden-city-pot-mom-pleads-no-contest-exchange-probation#stream/0.

Johannigman, Suzanne, and Valerie Eschiti. "Medical Use of Marijuana in Palliative Care." *Clinical Journal of Oncology Nursing* 17, no. 4 (July 30, 2013): 360–62. https://doi.org/10.1188/13.cjon.360-362.

Joseph, Andrew. "Marijuana Research Will Remain Restricted with DEA Decision." *STAT*, August 11, 2016. https://www.statnews.com/2016/08/10/marijuana-medical-research-dea/.

Josephson, Amelia. "The Cost of Living in Colorado." *SmartAsset*, August 15, 2016. https://smartasset.com/mortgage/the-cost-of-living-in-colorado.

Kahl, Matt. Interview with the author, May 10, 2017.

Kennedy, Bruce. "These 6 Groups Help Vets Get Access to Medical Marijuana." *Cannabist*, May 26, 2017. http://www.thecannabist.co/2017/05/26/veterans-medical-marijuana-nonprofit-military-ptsd/80228/.

Kershner, Isabel. "Israel, a Medical Marijuana Pioneer, Is Eager to Capitalize." *New York*

Times, December 17, 2016. https://www.nytimes.com/2016/12/17/world/middleeast/israel-a-medical-marijuana-pioneer-is-eager-to-capitalize.html?mcubz=2.

Kloosterman, Karin. "Dr. 'Cannabis': Alan Shackelford Puts Medicine into Marijuana, in Israel." *Green Prophet*, January 20, 2015. https://www.greenprophet.com/2015/01/dr-cannabis-alan-shackelford-puts-medicine-into-cannabis-in-israel/.

Knoss, Trent. "CU Boulder Researchers Receive State Grant to Study High-Potency Marijuana Effects." *CU Boulder Today*, December 16, 2016. http://www.colorado.edu/today/2016/12/16/cu-boulder-researchers-receive-state-grant-study-high-potency-marijuana-effects.

Knupp, Kelly. Interview with the author, June 13, 2017.

Koerner, Claudia. "Veteran with PTSD Faces Up to Life in Prison for Growing Marijuana." *BuzzFeed*. July 6, 2015. https://www.buzzfeed.com/claudiakoerner/veteran-with-ptsd-faces-up-to-life-in-prison-for-growing-mar?utm_term=.dppGJyZ0V#.yc6LmVzWq.

Kossen, Jeremy. "How Does Cannabis Consumption Affect Autism?" *Leafly*, May 19, 2016. Accessed January 29, 2017. https://www.leafly.com/news/health/how-does-cannabis-consumption-affect-autism.

KPS 4 Parents. "Parents in Crisis Can Be Vulnerable to Predators." *Making Special Education Actually Work*, December 12, 2013. http://blog.kps4parents.org/?p=1057.

Kreutter, Danielle. "New Law Requires Schools to Adopt a Medical Marijuana Policy." KKTV. June 6, 2016. http://www.kktv.com/content/news/New-Law-Requires-Schools-to-Adopt-a-Medical-Marijuana-Policy-382047851.html (accessed May 7, 2017).

Krogstad, Jens Manuel, and Jynnah Radford. "Key Facts About Refugees to the U.S." Pew Research Center. January 30, 2017. http://www.pewresearch.org/fact-tank/2017/01/30/key-facts-about-refugees-to-the-u-s/.

Lanahan, Leslie, and Micheal (producers). *Haze*. Trailer. June 28, 2013. https://www.youtube.com/watch?v=E1G2JX5IXks.

Lankenau, Stephen, Ekaterina Fedorova, Salini Mohanty, Chaka Dodson, Meghan Treese, Miles McNeeley, Carolyn Wong, and Ellen Iverson. "Young Adult Medical Marijuana Patients: Health Histories and Motives for Marijuana Use." 143rd American Public Health Association Annual Meeting and Exposition (APHA 2015), November 3, 2015. https://apha.confex.com/apha/143am/webprogram/Paper329467.html.

Laslo, Matt. "How the Pot Movement Changed in 2018." *Rolling Stone*, December 24, 2018. https://www.rollingstone.com/culture/culture-features/marijuana-weed-2018-changed-pot-772473/.

Lee, Martin A. *Smoke Signals: A Social History of Marijuana—Medical, Recreational, and Scientific.* New York: Scribner's, 2012.

_____. "Synthetic vs. Whole Plant CBD." *Medical Marijuana*, February 22, 2015. https://www.projectcbd.org/article/synthetic-vs-whole-plant-cbd.

"Legality of Cannabis by Country." Wikipedia. April 16, 2017. https://en.wikipedia.org/wiki/Legality_of_cannabis_by_country.

Levin, Sam. "Expots: Medical Marijuana Draws Parents to US for Their Children's Treatments." *The Guardian*, May 9, 2016. https://www.theguardian.com/society/2016/may/09/medical-marijuana-families-move-to-colorado-epilepsy.

Lindsey, Nick. "More Than 200,000 People Moved to Colorado Between 2013–2014." *Green Rush Daily*, October 15, 2015. https://www.greenrushdaily.com/2015/10/15/200000-people-moved-to-colorado/.

Lopez, German. "House Protects Marijuana Patients from Feds." *Vox*, May 30, 2014. https://www.vox.com/2014/5/30/5763654/the-house-just-voted-to-protect-medical-marijuana-patients-from.

Lubell, Maayan, and Lianne Back. "Israel Looks to Leverage Tech in $50 Billion Medical

Marijuana Market." Reuters. March 23, 2017. http://www.reuters.com/article/us-israel-cannabis-idUSKBN16U1PZ.

Maa, Edward, and Paige Figi. "The Case for Medical Marijuana in Epilepsy." *Epilepsia* 55, no. 6 (2014): 783–786.

Mack, Alison, and Janet E. Joy. *Marijuana as Medicine?: the Science Beyond the Controversy.* Washington, D.C.: National Academy, 2001.

Malloy, Daniel. "Meet the Last Georgia Medical Marijuana Refugees in Colorado." *Atlanta Journal Constitution.*, November 13, 2015. http://politics.blog.ajc.com/2015/11/13/meet-the-last-georgia-medical-marijuana-refugees-in-colorado/.

MAPS. "Marijuana for Symptoms of PTSD in U.S. Veterans." http://www.maps.org/research/mmj/marijuana-us.

"Marijuana Businesses Access to Banking Act of 2015 (2015—H.R. 2076)." GovTrack.us. https://www.govtrack.us/congress/bills/114/hr2076.

"Marijuana Plant Gives Choctaw Teen Chance at New Life." *Red Dirt Report.* December 17, 2014. http://www.reddirtreport.com/red-dirt-news/marijuana-plant-gives-choctaw-teen-chance-new-life.

Marijuana Policy Project. "Jared Polis Archives." MPP Blog. https://blog.mpp.org/tag/jared-polis/.

_____. "State Laws." https://www.mpp.org.

Marso, Andy. "Charges Against Garden City Mother Enflame Cannabis Community." Kansas Health Institute. June 9, 2015. http://www.khi.org/news/article/charges-against-garden-city-mother-enflame-cannabis-community.

Maule, W.J. "Medical Uses of Marijuana (Cannabis Sativa): Fact or Fallacy?" *British Journal of Biomedical Science* 72, no. 2 (January 2015): 85–91. https://doi.org/10.1080/09674845.2015.11666802.

Mawer, Rudy. "The Ketogenic Diet 101: A Beginner's Guide." *Healthline,* June 17, 2017. https://www.healthline.com/nutrition/ketogenic-diet-101.

Mayo Clinic. "Crohn's Disease." http://www.mayoclinic.org/diseases-conditions/crohns-disease/diagnosis-treatment/treatment/txc-20342074.

_____. "Fibromyalgia." September 8, 2016. http://www.mayoclinic.org/diseases-conditions/fibromyalgia/basics/definition/con-20019243.

McQuillan, Laura. "Kiwis Are Literally Dying to Use Medicinal Cannabis. Is a Change to the System Bold Enough?" stuff.co.nz. June 2, 2017. http://www.stuff.co.nz/national/93284426/kiwis-are-literally-dying-to-use-medicinal-cannabis-is-a-change-to-the-system-bold-enough.

Mcvay, Doug. "MedicalCannabis.Com: A Project of Patients out of Time." January 12, 2017. http://www.medicalcannabis.com/.

"Med Students Support Legal Marijuana." http://www.ucdenver.edu/academics/colleges/medicalschool/administration/news/ResearchNews/Pages/Med-Students-Support-Legal-Marijuana.aspx.

Migoya, David, and Allison Sherry. "Banks Given the Go-Ahead on Working with Marijuana Businesses." *Denver Post*, October 2, 2016. http://www.denverpost.com/2014/02/14/banks-given-the-go-ahead-on-working-with-marijuana-businesses/.

Military.com. "Traumatic Brain Injury Overview." http://www.military.com/benefits/veterans-health-care/traumatic-brain-injury-overview.html.

Minton, Mark. "Banda Pleads Not Guilty; Medical Cannabis Experts Testify." *Garden City Telegram*, April 7, 2017. http://www.gctelegram.com/62e6748c-d9bd-5cfd-b900-c1516afebccf.html.

_____. "Banda Sentenced to 12 Months Probation." *Garden City Telegram*, October 13, 2017. http://www.gctelegram.com/news/20171013/banda-sentenced-to-12-months-probation.

Mitchell, Thomas. "Colorado Board of Health Rejects PTSD as MMJ Condition." *Westword*, April 2, 2016. http://www.westword.com/news/colorado-board-of-health-rejects-ptsd-as-mmj-condition-6915169.

_____. "John Hickenlooper Signs Law Making PTSD Official Medical Marijuana Condition." *Westword*, June 8, 2017. http://www.westword.com/marijuana/ptsd-now-treatable-by-medical-marijuana-in-colorado-9132084.

_____. "Long Odds for Reintroduced Marijuana Banking Bill." *Westword*, April 2, 2016. http://www.westword.com/news/long-odds-for-reintroduced-marijuana-banking-bill-6674809.

Montopoli, Brian. "Does the Pot Pill Work?" *CBS News*. August 3, 2009. http://www.cbsnews.com/news/does-the-pot-pill-work/.

Moraff, Christopher. "The UN's Prohibitionism Impedes Drug Policy Reform." *Al Jazeera America*. March 17, 2015. http://america.aljazeera.com/opinions/2015/3/the-uns-prohibitionist-stance-impedes-drug-policy-reform.html.

Morris, Chris. "10 Top-Rated States for Medical Marijuana." CNBC. February 19, 2016. http://www.cnbc.com/2016/02/19/10-top-rated-states-for-medical-marijuana.html.

Moving for Marijuana. http://movingformarijuana.com/.

Mueller, Benjamin. "Using Data to Make Sense of a Racial Disparity in NYC Marijuana Arrests." *New York Times*, May 13, 2018. https://www.nytimes.com/2018/05/13/insider/data-marijuana-arrests-racial-disparity.html.

Mueller, Benjamin, Robert Gebeloff and Sahil Chinoy. "Surest Way to Face Marijuana Charges in New York: Be Black or Hispanic." *New York Times*, May 13, 2018. https://www.nytimes.com/2018/05/13/nyregion/marijuana-arrests-nyc-race.html?action=click&module=RelatedCoverage&pgtype=Article&region=Footer.

Mukherjee, Sy. "Here's Why This Marijuana Drug Company's Stock Is Soaring Today." *Fortune*, June 27, 2016. http://fortune.com/2016/06/27/gw-pharma-cannabis-drug-results/.

_____. "This Company Made the First FDA Approved, Marijuana Based Drug. Here's What It Wants to Do Next." *Fortune*, June 27, 2018. http://fortune.com/2018/06/27/fda-marijuana-gw-pharma-epidiolex-whats-next/

Mullin, Rick. "Cost to Develop New Pharmaceutical Drug Now Exceeds $2.5B." *Scientific American*, November 24, 2014. https://www.scientificamerican.com/article/cost-to-develop-new-pharmaceutical-drug-now-exceeds-2–5b/.

Murray, Jon. "Denver Council Deadlocks on New Marijuana Industry Caps." April 11, 2016. http://www.denverpost.com/2016/04/11/denver-council-deadlocks-on-new-marijuana-industry-caps/.

Narang, S., D. Gibson, A.D. Wasan, E.L. Ross, E. Michna, S.S. Nedeljkovic, and R.N. Jamison. "Efficacy of Dronabinol as an Adjuvant Treatment for Chronic Pain Patients on Opioid Therapy." *Journal of Pain: Official Journal of the American Pain Society* (March 2008). https://www.ncbi.nlm.nih.gov/pubmed/18088560.

National Academies of Sciences, Engineering, and Medicine. *The Health Effects of Cannabis and Cannabinoids: The Current State of Evidence and Recommendations for Research*. January 12, 2017. https://doi.org/10.17226/24625.

National Center for Natural Products Research. https://pharmacy.olemiss.edu/ncnpr/research-programs/cannabis-research/.

National Conference of State Legislatures. "State Medical Marijuana Laws." Updated August 1, 2019. http://www.ncsl.org/research/health/state-medical-marijuana-laws.aspx.

National Institutes of Health. "Genetic and Rare Diseases Information Center." https://rarediseases.info.nih.gov/diseases.

National Institute on Drug Abuse. "Drug Facts: Marijuana." Revised June 2018. https://www.drugabuse.gov/publications/drugfacts/marijuana.

_____. "NIDA's Role in Providing Marijuana for Research." March 20, 2017. https://www.drugabuse.gov/drugs-abuse/marijuana/nidas-role-in-providing-marijuana-research.

_____. "Overdose Death Rates." Revised August 2018. https://www.drugabuse.gov/related-topics/trends-statistics/overdose-death-rates.

National Jewish Health. "Colorado Marijuana Users Health Cohort." https://www.nationaljewish.org/clinical-trials/colorado-marijuana-users-health-cohort.

National Organization for the Reform of Marijuana Laws. "Working to Reform Marijuana Laws." http://norml.org/legal/medical-marijuana-2.

Newton, David. *Marijuana: A Reference Handbook.* ABC-CLIO, 2013. http://www.myilibrary.com?ID=45362.

"Nidal Hasan." Wikipedia. https://en.wikipedia.org/wiki/Nidal_Hasan (accessed May 22, 2017).

NIH (National Cancer Institute). "Cannabis and Cannabinoids." December 8, 2016. https://www.cancer.gov/about-cancer/treatment/cam/hp/cannabis-pdq#section/_11.

Nischal, Anil, Adarsh Tripathi, Anuradha Nischal, and J.K. Trivedi. "Suicide and Antidepressants: What Current Evidence Indicates." *Mens Sana Monographs* 10, no. 1 (January–December 2012): 33–44. https://www.ncbi.nlm.nih.gov/pmc/articles/PMC3353604/.

Nolin, Pierre Claude, Colin Kenny, and Senate Special Committee on Illegal Drugs. *Cannabis: Report of the Senate Special Committee on Illegal Drugs.* Toronto: University of Toronto Press, 2003.

Noonan, David. "Scientists Want the Smoke to Clear on Medical Marijuana Research." *Scientific American.* https://www.scientificamerican.com/article/scientists-want-the-smoke-to-clear-on-medical-marijuana-research/.

Odabasi, Mehmet. "Decriminalizing Marijuana: Understanding Marijuana Debate Through History and Policy." *European Scientific Journal* 10, no. 1 (January 2014). https://eujournal.org/index.php/esj/article/view/2545/2405.

Ogbru, Annette. "Benzodiazepines." RXList. May 2, 2016. http://www.rxlist.com/benzodiazepines/drugs-condition.htm.

Olinger, David "Kansas Holds Children of Colorado Veteran Who Uses Medical Marijuana." *Denver Post*, October 2, 2016. http://www.denverpost.com/2016/01/13/kansas-holds-children-of-colorado-veteran-who-uses-medical-marijuana/.

Ornstein, Charles. "Doctors Earn $3.5 Billion in Kickbacks from Pharmaceutical Companies." *Health Impact News*, October 3, 2014. https://healthimpactnews.com/2014/doctors-earn-3-5-billion-in-kickbacks-from-pharmaceutical-companies/.

Parents 4 Pot. "Wisconsin Advocates Push for Whole Plant Cannabis at CBD-Only Hearing." http://www.parents4pot.org/wisconsin_advocates_push#.WPemMlPyvBJ.

Park, Eileen. "NC Families Uproot Lives to Seek Medical Marijuana in Colorado." *WNCN News.* May 16, 2014. http://wncn.com/2014/05/16/nc-families-uproot-lives-to-seek-medical-marijuana-in-colorado/.

Pasquariello, Alex. "Cannabis Industry Org Forms to 'Be Ready' for National Legalization." *Cannabist*, June 16, 2017. http://www.thecannabist.co/2017/06/16/national-association-of-cannabis-businesses-marijuana-industry/81746/.

Peake, Gage. "Congress Pushes to Renew Rohrabacher-Farr Patient Protections." *Leafly*, April 11, 2017. https://www.leafly.com/news/politics/congress-pushes-renew-rohrabacher-farr-patient-protections.

Perlmutter, Ed. "Text—H.R.2652–113th Congress (2013–2014): Marijuana Businesses Access to Banking Act of 2013." Congress.gov. September 13, 2013. https://www.congress.gov/bill/113th-congress/house-bill/2652/text.

"Peter Dunne Says Medical Cannabis in Tragic Alex Renton Case Was Worthwhile." stuff.co.nz. July 2, 2015. http://www.stuff.co.nz/national/health/69888664/nelson-teenager-alex-renton-dies-despite-treatment-with-medical-cannabis.

Pharmacyte Biotech, Inc. "PharmaCyte Biotech Discusses Future of Cannabis Research Program, Competitors and More with Program's Director." *GlobeNewswire*, April 18, 2017. https://globenewswire.com/news-release/2017/04/18/961697/0/en/PharmaCyte-Biotech-Discusses-Future-of-Cannabis-Research-Program-Competitors-and-More-with-Program-s-Director.html.

Philipps, Dave. "Suicide Rate Among Veterans Has Risen Sharply Since 2001." *New York Times*, July 7, 2016. https://www.nytimes.com/2016/07/08/us/suicide-rate-among-veterans-has-risen-sharply-since-2001.html.

Phillips, Zach. Interview with the author, May 19, 2017.

Pierce, Lindsay. *Desperate Journey*. Trailer. Vimeo. February 4, 2017. https://vimeo.com/114290732.

Pletka, Vicki. Interview with the author, May 9, 2016.

Pollack, Andrew. "Marijuana-Based Drug Found to Reduce Epileptic Seizures." *New York Times*, March 15, 2016. https://www.nytimes.com/2016/03/15/business/marijuana-based-drug-found-to-reduce-epileptic-seizures.html?_r=0.

"Pot for PTSD? Colorado Reconsiders Medical Marijuana Rule." *CBS News*. July 15, 2015. http://www.cbsnews.com/news/pot-for-ptsd-colorado-reconsiders-medical-marijuana-rule/.

Press, Craig A., Kelly G. Knupp, and Kevin E. Chapman. "Parental Reporting of Response to Oral Cannabis Extracts for Treatment of Refractory Epilepsy." *Epilepsy and Behavior* 45 (2015): 49–52. https://doi.org/10.1016/j.yebeh.2015.02.043.

Preston, Caroline. "Parents Face Child Abuse Investigations Over Pot Use." *Al Jazeera America*. September 7, 2015. http://america.aljazeera.com/articles/2015/9/7/parents-face-child-abuse-investigations-over-marijuana-use.html.

ProCon. "History of Marijuana as Medicine: 2900 BC to Present." Updated on January 30, 2017. http://medicalmarijuana.procon.org/view.timeline.php?timelineID=000026.

_____. "Should Marijuana Be a Medical Option?" http://medicalmarijuana.procon.org/view.additional-resource.php?resourceID=000149.

_____. "10 Pharmaceutical Drugs Based on Cannabis" http://medicalmarijuana.procon.org/view.resource.php?resourceID=000883.

"PTSD: A Growing Epidemic." *NIH MedlinePlus the Magazine* (Winter 2009). https://medlineplus.gov/magazine/issues/winter09/articles/winter09pg10–14.html.

Pullen, Sara Marie. "What Are Cannabinoids?" *Leaf Science*, October 23, 2015. http://www.leafscience.com/2015/10/23/cannabinoids/.

Rahn, Bailey. "Cannabinoids 101: What Makes Cannabis Medicine?" *Leafly*, January 22, 2014. https://www.leafly.com/news/cannabis-101/cannabinoids-101-what-makes-cannabis-medicine.

_____. "What Is THCA and What Are the Benefits of This Cannabinoid?" *Leafly*, March 17, 2015. https://www.leafly.com/news/cannabis-101/what-is-thca-and-what-are-the-benefits-of-this-cannabinoid.

Realm of Caring. https://www.theroc.us/.

Reece, Kevin. "Medical Refugees Leave Texas for Marijuana Treatments." *KHOU News*. November 11, 2015. http://www.khou.com/news/health/medical-refugees-leave-texas-for-marijuana-treatments/55453259.

Reed, Danny. "What Does Trump AG Pick William Barr Mean for the Cannabis Industry?" *MG*, December 13, 2018. https://mgretailer.com/cannabis-news/what-does-trump-ag-pick-william-barr-mean-for-cannabis-industry/.

Rees, Gloria Van. "Woman with Terminal Cancer Jailed over Medication in Her System." KAKE.com. May 3, 2017. http://www.kake.com/story/35335390/woman-with-terminal-cancer-jailed-over-medication-in-her-system.

Riddle, Sierra. Interview with the author, September 21, 2017.

Rieder, Michael J. "Is the Medical Use of Cannabis a Therapeutic Option for Children?" *Paediatrics and Child Health* 21, no. 1 (January 2016): 1–5.

Riggs, Mike. "Obama's War on Pot." *The Nation*, June 29, 2015. https://www.thenation.com/article/obamas-war-pot/.

Roberts, Michael. "Inside Medical Marijuana Lawsuit Filed Against Colorado by Vets with PTSD." *Westword*, April 3, 2017. http://www.westword.com/news/inside-medical-marijuana-lawsuit-filed-against-colorado-by-vets-with-ptsd-7728656.

_____. "Remembering Jack Splitt: MMJ Jack's Law Namesake Loses Fight for Life." *Westword*, August 26, 2016. http://www.westword.com/news/remembering-jack-splitt-mmj-jacks-law-namesake-loses-fight-for-life-7982321.

Robinson, Melia. "Here's How Much Marijuana It Would Take to Kill You." *Business Insider*, November 5, 2016. http://www.businessinsider.com/can-marijuana-kill-you-2016-11.

Robnett, Teri. Interview with the author, February 17, 2017.

Rockoff, Jonathan D. "Mylan Faces Scrutiny Over Epipen Price Increases." *Wall Street Journal*, August 24, 2016. https://www.wsj.com/articles/mylan-faces-scrutiny-over-epipen-price-increases-1472074823.

Roffman, Roger. *Marijuana Nation: One Man's Chronicle of America Getting High*. New York: Pegasus, 2015.

Rohrabacher, Dana. "H.Amdt.748 to H.R.4660–113th Congress (2013–2014)." Congress.gov. May 30, 2014. https://www.congress.gov/amendment/113th-congress/house-amendment/748.

Rollins, Judy A. "Pot for Tots: Children and Medical Marijuana." *Pediatric Nursing* 40, no. 2 (March–April 2014): 59–60.

Root, Sue. Interview with the author, May 10, 2016.

"Rose Renton Petition for Medical Cannabis." *NORML New Zealand*. March 22, 2016. https://norml.org.nz/2016/sign-the-rose-renton-petition-for-medicinal-cannabis/.

Rosen, Liana W. *International Drug Control Policy: Background and U.S. Responses*. March 16, 2015. https://fas.org/sgp/crs/row/RL34543.pdf.

Rough, Lisa. "Can You Legally Transport Cannabis Across State Lines?" *Leafly*, June 23, 2017. https://www.leafly.com/news/cannabis-101/can-you-transport-cannabis-between-two-legal-states.

Russo, Ethan B. "Taming THC: Potential Cannabis Synergy and Phytocannabinoid-Terpenoid Entourage Effects." *British Journal of Pharmacology* 163, no. 7 (2011): 1344–1364. PMC. https://doi.org/10.1111/j.1476–5381.2011.01238.x.

"S. 683 (114th): Compassionate Access, Research Expansion, and Respect States Act of 2015." GovTrack.us. https://www.govtrack.us/congress/bills/114/s683/summary.

Safer Lock. "The Secret Danger for Parents Who Smoke Medical Marijuana." December 9, 2015. https://saferlockrx.com/the-secret-danger-for-parents-who-smoke-medical-marijuana/.

Sanchez, Amanda. Interview with the author, May 10, 2016.

Sanchez, Steve. Interview with the author, May 10, 2016.

Schou, Nick. "PTSD-Stricken Marine Vet Faces Five Years in Oklahoma Prison for Growing Six Marijuana Plants." *OC Weekly*, March 8, 2017. http://www.ocweekly.com/news/ptsd-stricken-marine-vet-faces-five-years-in-oklahoma-prison-for-growing-six-marijuana-plants-7493535.

Schuba, Tom, "Cannabis 101: A Guide to Medical Marijuana in Illinois." *Chicago Sun Times*, September 5, 2018. https://chicago.suntimes.com/cannabis/illinois-medical-marijuana-law-dispensaries-cannabis/.

Schulte, Brigid. "Mom Who Uses Medical Marijuana Faces Up to 30 Years in Prison." *Washington Post*, June 8, 2015. https://www.washingtonpost.com/news/local/wp/2015/

06/08/mom-who-uses-medical-marijuana-faces-up-to-30-years-in-prison/?utm_term=.b4fdf8f44e3f.

Schwartz, Yardena. "The Holy Land of Medical Marijuana." USNews.com, April 11, 2017. https://www.usnews.com/news/best-countries/articles/2017–04–11/israel-is-a-global-leader-in-marijuana-research.

"Scientists to Government: Make It Easier to Study Marijuana." *New York Times*, January 17, 2017. https://www.nytimes.com/2017/01/17/opinion/scientists-to-government-make-it-easier-to-study-marijuana.html?mcubz=2.

Sederberg, Vicente. "Vicente Sederberg LLC—The Marijuana Law-Firm." 2016. http://vicentesederberg.com/.

Sensible Colorado. "History of Colorado's Marijuana Laws." http://sensiblecolorado.org/history-of-co-medical-marijuana-laws/.

Senthilingam, Meera. "Germany Joins Global Experiment on Marijuana Legalization." CNN.com. March 6, 2017. http://www.cnn.com/2016/12/29/health/global-marijuana-cannabis-laws/index.html.

Shackelford, Alan. Interview with the author, June 20, 2016.

Shane, Leo, and Patricia Kime. "New VA Study Finds 20 Veterans Commit Suicide Each Day." *Military Times*, July 7, 2016. http://www.militarytimes.com/story/veterans/2016/07/07/va-suicide-20-daily-research/86788332/.

Sherman, Erik. "Nixon's Drug War, an Excuse to Lock up Blacks and Protesters, Continues." *Forbes*, March 23, 2016. http://www.forbes.com/sites/eriksherman/2016/03/23/nixons-drug-war-an-excuse-to-lock-up-blacks-and-protesters-continues/#7e07c98a5099.

Simmons, Kate McKee. "Colorado Reports $1.3 Billion in Marijuana Sales in 2016." *Westword*, May 30, 2017. http://www.westword.com/marijuana/colorado-reports-13-billion-in-marijuana-sales-in-2016–8785295.

Sloman, Larry. *Reefer Madness: The History of Marijuana in America*. Indianapolis: Bobbs-Merrill, 1979.

Smith, Aaron. "10 Things to Know About Legal Pot." *CNNMoney*. May 26, 2017. http://money.cnn.com/2017/04/19/news/legal-marijuana-420/index.html.

Smith, Phillip. "Mother Who Used Medical Cannabis to Treat Deadly Disease Had Her Son Taken Away, Faces 28 Years in Prison." *Alternet*. http://www.alternet.org/drugs/shona-banda-medical-marijuana-legal-nightmare-continues.

Solé, Elise. "Wisconsin Family to Move to Colorado So Daughter, 4, Has Access to Marijuana." *Yahoo! News*, April 23, 2015. https://www.yahoo.com/news/wisconsin-family-to-move-to-colorado-so-daughter-117202093802.html.

Staver, Matthew. "Marijuana Refugees Face Real Estate Challenges." *Health Care*. CNBC. February 20, 2014. http://www.cnbc.com/2014/02/04/marijuana-refugees-face-real-estate-challenges.html.

Stein, Perry. "Veterans Drop Hundreds of Empty Pill Bottles in Front of the White House." *Washington Post*, November 11, 2015. https://www.washingtonpost.com/news/local/wp/2015/11/11/veterans-drop-hundreds-of-empty-pill-bottles-in-front-of-the-white-house/?utm_term=.f86ca9ca51d4.

Stern, Ray. "First Marijuana Testing for Vets with PTSD Underway in Phoenix; Volunteers Wanted." *Phoenix New Times*, May 31, 2017. http://www.phoenixnewtimes.com/news/first-marijuana-testing-for-vets-with-ptsd-underway-in-phoenix-volunteers-wanted-9072949.

Stormes, Jennie. "Cannabis RN." http://www.jenniestormesrn.com/cannabis-rn-blog.html.

_____. Interview with the author, May 2, 2016.

Strasser, Franz (producer). "Lancaster, Pennsylvania: America's Refugee Capital." *BBC*

News. January 27, 2017. http://www.bbc.com/news/av/world-us-canada-38776233/the-refugee-capital-of-the-us.

Sullum, Jacob. "Congress Did Not Legalize Medical Marijuana." *Forbes,* January 5, 2016. https://www.forbes.com/sites/jacobsullum/2015/12/31/congress-did-not-legalize-medical-marijuana/#2ced8f933a4d.

Szalavitz, Maia. "Marijuana: The Next Diabetes Drug?" *Time,* May 21, 2013. http://healthland.time.com/2013/05/21/marijuana-the-next-diabetes-drug/.

Taylor, Stuart S. "Marijuana Policy and Presidential Leadership: How to Avoid a Federal-State Train Wreck." Brookings. July 28, 2016. https://www.brookings.edu/research/marijuana-policy-and-presidential-leadership-how-to-avoid-a-federal-state-train-wreck/.

Thompson, Simon. "97% of Texas Marijuana Convictions Are for Possession." KRWG. http://krwg.org/post/97-texas-marijuana-convictions-are-possession.

Torres, Sandra. "Lily's Hope: Part 2: How Medical Marijuana Is Working in Colorado." *CBS 58.* July 16, 2015. http://www.cbs58.com/story/29568893/lilys-hope-part-2-how-medical-marijuana-is-working-in-colorado.

TraumaticBrainInjury.com. "Mild TBI Symptoms." http://www.traumaticbraininjury.com/symptoms-of-tbi/mild-tbi-symptoms/.

Treat, Lauren, Kevin E. Chapman, Kathryn L. Colborn, and Kelly G. Knupp. "Duration of Use of Oral Cannabis Extract in a Cohort of Pediatric Epilepsy Patients." *Epilepsia* 58, no. 1 (2016): 123–27. https://doi.org/10.1111/epi.13617.

Tress, Luke. "In Pioneering Study, Israeli Researchers Target Autism with Cannabis." *Times of Israel,* March 8, 2017. http://www.timesofisrael.com/in-pioneering-study-israeli-researchers-target-autism-with-cannabis/.

Turner, Coltyn. Interview with the author, May 11, 2016.

Turner, Wendy. Interview with the author, May 11, 2016.

Tvert, Mason. Interview with the author, January 19, 2017.

United Nations Office on Drugs and Crime. "The 1912 Hague International Opium Convention." https://www.unodc.org/unodc/en/frontpage/the-1912-hague-international-opium-convention.html.

United States Department of Justice. Memorandum for United States Attorneys. June 29, 2011. https://www.justice.gov/sites/default/files/oip/legacy/2014/07/23/dag-guidance-2011-for-medical-marijuana-use.pdf.

University of Colorado Denver School of Medicine. "Research." http://www.ucdenver.edu/academics/colleges/medicalschool/research/Pages/research.aspx.

University of Virginia. "Gordie's Story." https://gordiecenter.studenthealth.virginia.edu/gordie/gordies-story.

U.S. Department of Health and Human Services. "NIH Fact Sheets—Post-Traumatic Stress Disorder (PTSD)." National Institutes of Health. https://report.nih.gov/NIH-factsheets/ViewFactSheet.aspx?csid=58.

_____. "Parental Drug Use as Child Abuse." National Institutes of Health. https://www.childwelfare.gov/pubPDFs/drugexposed.pdf.

U.S. Department of State. "Refugee Admissions." https://www.state.gov/j/prm/ra/.

U.S. Department of Veterans Affairs. "How Common Is PTSD?" PTSD: National Center for PTSD. July 5, 2007. https://www.ptsd.va.gov/public/ptsd-overview/basics/how-common-is-ptsd.asp.

_____. "Marijuana Use and PTSD among Veterans." PTSD: National Center for PTSD. December 17, 2014. https://www.ptsd.va.gov/professional/co-occurring/marijuana_use_ptsd_veterans.asp.

U.S. Food and Drug Administration. "Current Good Manufacturing Practices (CGMP) for Drugs: Reports, Guidances and Additional Information." https://www.fda.gov/

drugs/developmentapprovalprocess/manufacturing/questionsandanswersoncurre-ntgoodmanufacturingpracticescgmpfordrugs/default.htm.

_____. "The Drug Development Process—Step 3: Clinical Research." https://www.fda.gov/ForPatients/Approvals/Drugs/ucm405622.htm (accessed June 25, 2017).

_____. "Marijuana Research with Human Subjects." https://www.fda.gov/newsevents/publichealthfocus/ucm421173.htm.

"USDOJ New Policy." October 19, 2009. http://medicalmarijuana.procon.org/sourcefiles/USDOJNewPolicy.pdf.

Veterans Cannabis Project. http://www.vetscp.org/#.

Vibrant Health Clinic. http://www.vibranthealthclinic.com/ (accessed January 29, 2017).

Vicente, Brian. Interview with the author, February 8, 2017.

"Vital Signs: Alcohol Poisoning Deaths—United States, 2010–2012." *Morbidity and Mortality Weekly Report*, 65, no. 53 (January 9, 2015): 1238–1242. https://www.cdc.gov/mmwr/preview/mmwrhtml/mm6353a2.htm?s_cid=mm6353a2_w.

Wack, Kevin. "Big Banks Worked with Pot Industry, Despite Denials, Records Show." *American Banker*, January 11, 2017. https://www.americanbanker.com/news/big-banks-worked-with-pot-industry-despite-denials-records-show.

Wagner, Angie. "Night of Partying Proves Deadly for Popular Student." *Los Angeles Times*, November 28, 2004. http://articles.latimes.com/2004/nov/28/news/adna-drinkdeath28/2.

Wagner, Peter, and Bernadette Rabuy. "Mass Incarceration: The Whole Pie, 2016." Prison Policy Initiative. March 14, 2016. https://www.prisonpolicy.org/reports/pie2016.html

Wallace, Alicia. "America's Marijuana Industry Headed for $24 Billion by 2025." *Cannabist*, February 22, 2017. http://www.thecannabist.co/2017/02/22/report-united-states-marijuana-sales-projections-2025/74059/.

_____. "How Colorado Became the Planet's Top Mentor in Legalizing and Regulating Cannabis." *Cannabist*, October 25, 2016. http://www.thecannabist.co/2016/10/25/colorado-marijuana-mentor-states-international-legalization/65868/.

_____. "Medical Marijuana Could Poach More Than $4B from Pharma Sales Annually." *Cannabist*, May 24, 2017. http://www.thecannabist.co/2017/05/24/medical-marijuana-pharmaceutical-sales-impact/80045/.

_____. "New Federal Bill Would Allow Banking for Marijuana Businesses." *Cannabist*, April 27, 2017. http://www.thecannabist.co/2017/04/27/federal-marijuana-banking-bill-congress-perlmutter/78531/.

Walsh, Zach, Robert Callaway, Lynne Belle-Isle, Rielle Capler, Robert Kay, Philippe Lucas, and Susan Holtzman. "Cannabis for Therapeutic Purposes: Patient Characteristics, Access, and Reasons for Use." *International Journal of Drug Policy* 24, no. 6 (November 2013): 511–16. https://doi.org/10.1016/j.drugpo.2013.08.010.

Waltz, Vanessa. "Interview: Jason Cranford on Haleigh's Hope, Colorado Medical Cannabis Laws, and the Realm of Caring Waiting List." *Ladybud*. April 2, 2014. http://www.ladybud.com/2014/04/02/interview-jason-cranford-on-haleighs-hope-colorado-medical-cannabis-laws-and-the-realm-of-caring-waiting-list/.

Ware, M.A., and D. Ziemianski. "Medical Education on Cannabis and Cannabinoids: Perspectives, Challenges, and Opportunities." *Clinical Pharmacology and Therapeutics* 97, no. 6 (May 22, 2015): 548–50. https://doi.org/10.1002/cpt.103.

Warner, Joel. "Charlotte's Web: Untangling One of Colorado's Biggest Cannabis Success Stories." *Westword*, May 21, 2016. http://www.westword.com/news/charlottes-web-untangling-one-of-colorados-biggest-cannabis-success-stories-6050830.

Washburn, Polly. "Public Support for Medical and Recreational Marijuana Legalization Hits All-Time High." *Cannabist*, August 8, 2017. http://www.thecannabist.co/2017/08/08/marijuana-legalization-opinion-poll-americans/85562/.

"Washington Considers Allowing Medical Marijuana in Schools." *Cannabist*. http://www.thecannabist.co/2017/01/17/medical-marijuana-schools-washington/71550/.

Watkins, Eli. "Pot Activists Have Been Holding Their Breath for Months on Jeff Sessions." CNN. June 17, 2017. http://www.cnn.com/2017/06/17/politics/jeff-sessions-marijuana/index.html.

Watson, Elaine. "What Is the Regulatory Status of CBD in Food and Beverage Products?" *Food navigator-usa.com*, October 10, 2018. https://www.foodnavigator-usa.com/Article/2018/10/11/SPECIAL-FEATURE-What-is-the-regulatory-status-of-CBD-in-food-and-beverage-products.

Watts, Lindsay. "Disabled JeffCo Student's Cannabis Medication Confiscated, School Cites Federal Law." *Denver Channel*, February 10, 2015. http://www.thedenverchannel.com/news/local-news/marijuana/disabled-jeffco-students-cannabis-medication-confiscated-school-cites-federal-law.

Weed for Warriors Project. http://www.wfwproject.org/.

"Weed Warrior Kris Lewandowski No Longer Faces Life in Prison." *GFarma News*, June 8, 2017. http://gfarma.news/entertainment-news/weed-warrior-kris-lewandowski-no-longer-faces-life-prison/.

Wegman, Jesse. "The Injustice of Marijuana Arrests." *New York Times*, July 28, 2014. https://www.nytimes.com/2014/07/29/opinion/high-time-the-injustice-of-marijuana-arrests.html?mcubz=2.

Whaley, Monte. "Colorado Districts Wrestle with New Law Allowing Students to Use Medical Marijuana at School." *Denver Post*, August 22, 2016. http://www.denverpost.com/2016/08/22/schools-medical-marijuana-jacks-law/.

"What Are Cannabinoids?" *Leaf Science*, February 1, 2017. http://www.leafscience.com/2015/10/23/cannabinoids/.

White, Daniel. "Court: DEA Must Stop Raids on Legal Medical Marijuana." *Time*, October 20, 2015. http://time.com/4080110/dea-medical-marijuana-california-ruling/.

Williams, Timothy. "Marijuana Arrests Outnumber Those for Violent Crimes, Study Finds." *New York Times*, October 12, 2016. https://www.nytimes.com/2016/10/13/us/marijuana-arrests.html?mcubz=2.

Willis, Carly. "Kansas Man Arrested After Growing Cannabis to Control Seizures." *KSNT News*. April 20, 2017. http://ksnt.com/2017/04/20/kansas-man-arrested-after-growing-cannabis-to-control-seizures/.

Wing, Nick. "Obama Explains Increasing Medical Marijuana Crackdowns, Raids in 'Rolling Stone' Interview." *Huffington Post*, April 25, 2012. http://www.huffingtonpost.com/2012/04/25/obama-marijuana-raids-rolling-stone_n_1451744.html.

Woo, Andrew. "June 2016 Colorado Rent Report—Apartment List." *Apartment List Rentonomics*, August 26, 2016. Acceshttps://www.apartmentlist.com/rentonomics/june-2016-colorado-apartment-list-rent-report/.

Woods, Lauren. "World's Top Researcher of Rare Genetic Liver Disease Coming to UConn Health." *UConn Today*, September 22, 2016. http://today.uconn.edu/2016/09/worlds-top-glycogen-storage-disease-program-coming-uconn-health/.

"Would You Risk Going to Jail to Ease Your Child's Suffering?" *Next*, October 23, 2015. http://www.nowtolove.co.nz/news/real-life/love-and-the-drug-6953 (accessed September 20, 2017).

Wyatt, Kristen. "Colorado House Gives Prelim OK to Lower Limit: 16 Marijuana Plants Per Residence." *Cannabist*. http://www.thecannabist.co/2017/03/10/colorado-marijuana-plant-limit-home/75407/ (accessed September 20, 2017).

_____. "Colorado Lawmakers Call for Adding PTSD to Medical Pot List." *Cannabist*. http://www.thecannabist.co/2016/09/21/colorado-ptsd-medical-marijuana-qualifying-conditions-list/63599/.

_____. "Colorado Senate Committee Lowers Marijuana Plant Limit to 12, or 24 with Registration." *Cannabist.* http://www.thecannabist.co/2017/03/23/colorado-marijuana-plant-limit-bill/76003/.

Young, Saundra. "Marijuana Stops Child's Severe Seizures." CNN.com. August 7, 2013. http://www.cnn.com/2013/08/07/health/charlotte-child-medical-marijuana/index.html.

_____. "Medical Marijuana Refugees: 'This was our only hope.'" CNN.com. March 10, 2014. http://www.cnn.com/2014/03/10/health/medical-marijuana-refugees/.

_____. "3-Year-Old Is Focus of Medical Marijuana Battle." CNN.com. January 15, 2014. http://www.cnn.com/2014/01/15/health/cannabis-landon-riddle/index.html.

Zillow, Inc. "Colorado Home Prices and Home Values." https://www.zillow.com/co/home-values/.

Index

Numbers in **bold italics** indicate pages with illustrations

221